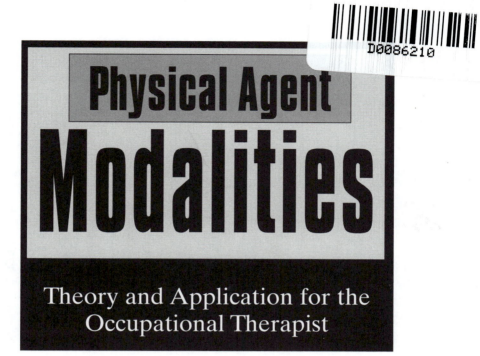

Physical Agent
Modalities

Theory and Application for the
Occupational Therapist

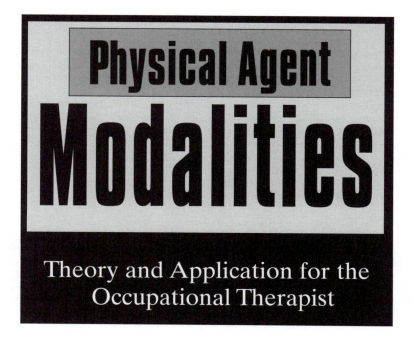

Physical Agent Modalities

Theory and Application for the Occupational Therapist

Alfred G. Bracciano, EdD, OTR

Saginaw Valley State University
Saginaw, MI

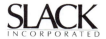

SLACK
INCORPORATED

6900 Grove Rd • Thorofare, NJ 08086

Publisher: John H. Bond
Editorial Director: Amy E. Drummond

The procedures and practices described in this book should be implemented in a manner consistent with the professional standards set for the circumstances that apply in each specific situation. Every effort has been made to confirm the accuracy of the information presented and to correctly relate generally accepted practices. The author, editor, and publisher cannot accept responsibility for errors or exclusions or for the outcome of the application of the material presented herein. There is no expressed or implied warranty of this book or information imparted by it.

Care has been taken to ensure that drug selection, dosages, and treatments are in accordance with currently accepted/recommended practice. Due to continuing research, changes in government policy and regulations, and various effects of drug reactions and interactions, it is recommended that the reader review all materials and literature provided for each drug, especially those that are new or not frequently used.

Any review or mention of specific companies or products is not intended as an endorsement by the author or the publisher.

The work SLACK publishes is peer reviewed. Prior to publication, recognized leaders in the field, educators, and clinicians provide important feedback on the concepts and content that we publish. We welcome feedback on this work.

Bracciano, Alfred
    Physical agent modalities : theory and application for the occupational therapist / Alfred Bracciano.
        p. ; cm.
    Includes bibliographical references and index.
    ISBN 1-55642-376-4 (alk. paper)
    1. Medicine, physical. 2. Physical therapy. 3. Occupational therapists. I. Title.
    [DNLM: 1. Occupational therapy--methods. 2. Cryotherapy. 3. Electric Stimulation Therapy. 4. Heat--therapeutic use. 5. Ultrasonic Therapy. WB 555 B796p 2000]
    RM700 .B68 2000
    615.8'2--dc21

                                                                                    00-025400

Printed in Canada.

Published by: SLACK Incorporated
                6900 Grove Road
                Thorofare, NJ 08086-9447 USA
                Telephone: 856-848-1000
                Fax: 856-853-5991
                www.slackbooks.com

Contact SLACK Incorporated for more information about other books in this field or about the availability of our books from distributors outside the United States.

Last digit is print number: 10   9   8   7   6   5   4   3   2   1

Dedication

To my wife Tamara, for her patience, love, and encouragement throughout this process. To my children, Christian, Elizabeth, Alfred, and Matthew, who thought my home office and computer were "my work" and who played numerous hours of Legos on the floor while I worked on the manuscript; to my father Alfred Sr., who modeled creativity and perseverence through his writing and work, and to my mother for her wisdom and support.

Contents

Acknowledgments

This book has evolved over a number of years, and as with any major project or life experience, there are a number of individuals who have influenced the outcome and impacted the final product. Certainly a major impetus in completing this text has been the the feedback and experiences of my students from Saginaw Valley State University who struggled to put physical agents into perspective following exposure to these modalities on their Level I and Level II Fieldwork. Clinicians and clinical faculty also called for a text written with an occupational therapy perspective which would assist them in more effectively incorporating physical agents into clinical practice. Their feedback, review, and encouragement have been invaluable. Special thanks to Kim Bartlett, OTR, for her illustrations and assistance in clarifying through art some of the concepts in the text; to Mr. David Czupinski, OTR, CHT for his assistance with the chapter on neuromuscular electrical stimulation; and to Lori Krantz, who always knew where to locate my references. Thanks also to Mr. Don Earley, MA, OTR, friend and colleague, for his work on superficial thermal agents, as well as for covering my classes when needed and for assisting with the pictures and presentations. My heartfelt thanks to Mark Griffin, Kristen Rievert, Tammy Schnell, Kourtney Willford, and Sara Schindehette for "modeling" for the pictures, and to all of my students who have helped develop this content through their questions.

Debra Toulson from SLACK Incorporated must be commended for keeping me on track and focused. Deb acted as the intermediary among all of the talented people from SLACK and made the publishing process, if not fun, at least somewhat less painful.

The individual who had the greatest influence on my professional career and who provided opportunities to expand and challenge me was Dr. Crystal M. Lange. Throughout her life, Dr. Lange exemplified the consummate scholar, administrator, clinician, and friend. Dr. Lange's support, encouragement, and unwavering confidence made it possible for me to think beyond my boundaries and limitations. Her life example as a transformational leader and her role as a mentor to me have provided a perspective and approach to life, and to our profession, which has been invaluable. She is sorely missed.

Finally, a very special and heartfelt thanks to my wife Tamara, who has pushed, prodded, and supported my work and this project through all these years. Her support, love, patience, and encouragement have made it possible to complete this project as we raised a family and underwent the myriad life experiences which challenge us every day. I could not have done this without her.

Alfred G. Bracciano, EdD, OTR

About the Author

Alfred G. Bracciano, EdD, OTR, is an occupational therapist who is a professor and founding chair of the occupational therapy program at Saginaw Valley State University in Saginaw, Michigan. In addition to his teaching responsibilities, Dr. Bracciano has a private practice with ancillary medical staff privileges at Huron Memorial Hospital in Bad Axe, Michigan, specializing in orthopedic injuries and general rehabilitation in a rural setting. Dr. Bracciano received his bachelor of science degree in occupational therapy from Wayne State University in Detroit, a master of science in administration degree from Central Michigan University, and a doctor of education from Western Michigan University in Kalamazoo, Michigan.

Dr. Bracciano has written a number of articles and chapters on physical agents and rural health issues, was a founding member of the editorial board for AOTA's *Innovations in Occupational Therapy Education*, serves as a reviewer for the *Journal of Rural Health*, and serves on the St. Mary's Hospital Institutional Review Board for research in Saginaw, Michigan. In addition to his publications, Dr. Bracciano has presented extensively on physical agent topics and orthopedic conditions related to occupational therapy practice. Dr. Bracciano has also served in a number of roles on the state level in the Michigan Occupational Therapy Association, including President, Vice President, Secretary, and Academic Chair for the Council on Education.

Contributing Authors

David Czupinski, OTR, CHT
Senior Therapist
St. John's Health Systems
Detroit, Michigan

Don Earley, MA, OTR
Assistant Professor
Occupational Therapy Department
Saginaw Valley State University
Saginaw, Michigan

Introduction

Physical Agent Modalities: Theory and Application for the Occupational Therapist grew out of my frustration in attempting to find a textbook related to physical agents which would be appropriate for my students at Saginaw Valley and which tied the potential benefits of physical agents to occupational performance. This text is a response to a need identified by our students at SVSU, and by clinical faculty and clinicians who have expressed the desire for a text to provide an overview of physical agents within clinical practice.

With managed care, health care delivery, and reimbursement driven with ever increasing frequency to outcome based criteria, occupational therapists are incorporating physical agents into clinical practice. Specialization and the growth in occupational therapists treating the demands of orthopedic and hand injuries have also contributed to the interest in and need for training and information related to physical agents. Many occupational therapists who use physical agents are criticized for their lack of education and training in use. Academic content in physical agents is not required as a part of the basic training and education in entry-level practice, and graduates may be unprepared to incorporate these agents into their practice. Other therapists using physical agents are trained on-the-job, through in-service, informal training, or through a weekend course. Though therapists may learn to safely apply physical agents through these methods, the profession and clinician have lacked a foundational text related to these physical agents. Occupational therapy clinicians have asked for a text to address their questions and concerns related to physical agents; this book is a response to their need.

Though clinicians have embraced physical agent technologies as part of clinical practice, there continues to be some controversy within the profession as to whether physical agents are truly occupational in nature. Being an academic as well as a clinician, I often feel as if I am a pariah when discussing physical agents as part of clinical practice with some of my colleagues in education. Part of the continuing controversy is due to the misperception that physical agents are used with *all* disabilities and supercede occupation. This could not be further from the truth. A thorough understanding of the healing process and an understanding of *how* physical agents work is vital to their correct and effective application. Additionally, physical agents in and of themselves are less effective unless paired with functional activity or occupation. Hopefully, with the publication of this text, further dialogue and understanding within the profession will occur.

This text is intended to provide the occupational therapist with basic foundational knowledge in the application and theory related to the most commonly used physical agents by occupational therapists. This text is not designed to be an all-inclusive scientific treatise on the basic sciences related to these agents. My position is that basic science content should be addressed in the primary science or foundational courses of physics, anatomy, biology, and others. The material and information presented is intended to explain the underlying theory and foundations of physical agents, and to relate how these agents can assist the occupational therapist in clinical practice by facilitating occupational performance and outcomes in our patients. Certainly, technologies and regulatory issues will continue to change and require clinicians to actively continue their education through reading, research, and workshops.

This text discusses the primary physical agents used by occupational therapists in clinical practice. Each chapter is formatted to provide the reader with the basic biophysiological principles of the physical agent, application of the agent, precautions and indications, and new terminology. A case study is included in some chapters to facilitate the clinical reasoning process for the clinician and to challenge their thinking. There are a variety of approaches to the conditions we treat as occupational therapists, and after review of this text, clinicians will have yet another technology and treatment approach which can be used to facilitate occupational function in our patients.

I hope that *Physical Agent Modalities: Theory and Application for the Occupational Therapist* provides you, the reader, with the information necessary to strengthen your clinical practice and to improve your effectiveness as an occupational therapist.

Chapter One

Regulatory Guidelines for the Use of Physical Agents

Learning Objectives

1. Discuss the professional issues related to physical agent use in occupational therapy.
2. Identify the challenges and changes in the health care system impacting the profession.
3. Discuss the ethical responsibilities in using physical agents.
4. Discuss the AOTA position on physical agent use and educational preparation.
5. Identify those states and regulatory agencies which govern the use of physical agents by occupational therapists.

Terminology

Competency	Physical agent modality
Entry-level practice	Regulatory
Ethics	Standards

Background

The profession of occupational therapy has evolved through a variety of internal and external forces impacting on clinical practice and theory development over the course of its existence. Recent changes to the United States health care system and to those professions providing services are directly impacting clinical practice for occupational therapists. The profession of occupational therapy has been challenged on all fronts: changes in Medicare and insurance reimbursement, managed care, the expanded scope of physical therapy practice to incorporate language and domain that was historically the realm of occupational therapy, questions regarding the efficacy of occupational therapy in the psychosocial realm, regulatory and competency issues raised by the National Board for Certification in Occupational Therapy (NBCOT), advances in technology, cost containment, and efficacy issues. A widely debated topic in occupational therapy, physical medicine, and rehabilitation in general has been the use of physical agent modalities (PAMs) or technologies in the treatment process, and the occupational therapist's role in using them. There have been proponents as well as critics for the use of physical agents within the practice of occupational therapy, though the dialogue between the competing positions has been less vociferous in recent years.

The American Occupational Therapy Association (AOTA) developed a Physical Agent Modality Task Force in 1990 to explore the issues related to physical agents and the philosophical positions of the involved constituencies. One aspect of the Task Force was to undertake a member data survey to determine specific use of physical agents. Therapists in private practice used modalities with greater frequency than those therapists in non mental health practice. Hot packs (44%), cold packs (42%), and paraffin (39%) were the modalities most frequently used by non mental health practitioners, followed by contrast baths (34%), electrical stimulation (28%) and fluidotherapy (22%). Therapists in private practice cited the use of electrical stimulation (45%), contrast baths (42%), ultrasound (32%), and whirlpool (32%) as more frequently used modalities.[1] The AOTA official policy statement concluded that physical agent modalities could be used as an adjunct to purposeful activity to enhance occupational performance,[2] but that the practice was not considered "entry-level". Many leaders of the profession, however, were opposed to the use of physical agents, believing them inconsistent with the profession's theory and philosophy of occupation. Taylor and Humphry[3] found that 80% of the 650 respondents in physical disability practice believed that the use of physical agents reflected a natural evolution of the profession toward new technologies, and a full 58% thought that the use of physical agents was consistent with the philosophical base of occupational therapy. Interestingly, the respondents who identified themselves as educators were less ardent than clinicians that physical agents should be taught as part of academic curricula. Other educators surveyed also disagreed with the inclusion of physical agents in clinical practice.[4]

Cornish-Painter, Peterson,[5] surveyed occupational therapists from the physical disabilities special interest section regarding their use of, education in, competency testing for, and opinion on eight physical agents. They found that the most common method of education in use of physical agents was through on-the-job training, and the least common was higher level accredited education. The AOTA's *A Guide for the Preparation of Occupational Therapy Practitioners for the Use of Physical Agent Modalities*[6] describes the base of information and knowledge necessary to use physical agents, the skill and experience needed, and the preparation spanning the therapists' career. AOTA's recommendations for appropriate mechanisms to obtain the requisite knowledge was through formal academic course work or continuing education. Cornish-Painter and Peterson's[5] survey found that the AOTA's recommendations were inconsistent with the most commonly reported methods used: informal on-the-job training, self-taught, or observations of physical therapists. Glauner, Ekes, et al's[7] study on the theoretical and technical competence and education of physical agents in occupational therapy practice found that the level and type of education needed to obtain competence in physical agent use varied widely and was dependent on the type of agent. Glauner and Ekes[7] also recommended that occupational therapy educational programs be provided a mechanism to ensure that content in physical agents would be developed. Funk[8] also reported that respondents in their study believed that entry-level occupational therapy programs should educate students in the use of PAMs.

There is an apparent incongruency between the desire of clinicians to obtain basic information regarding physical agents at an academic level and the reality of on-the-job training which is occurring. As greater numbers of occupational therapists and students completing fieldwork are exposed to and use physical agents as an adjunctive method to treatment, foundational information related to physical agents at an accredited educational level is vital to ensure safe application and integration with the philosophical tenets of occupational therapy.

Philosophical Issues

PAMs are defined as the interventions or technologies that produce a response in soft tissue through the use of light, water, temperature, sound, or electricity. PAMs include, but are not limited to: paraffin baths, cold packs, hot packs, fluidotherapy, contrast baths, ultrasound, whirlpool, electrical stimulation, neuromuscular stimulation (NMES), and transcutaneous electrical nerve stimulation (TENS).[9] The AOTA has advocated the use of physical agents as an adjunctive method used in preparation for or in conjunction with patient involvement in purposeful activity or occupation. These "adjunctive methods" support occupational performance components that allow the patient to participate in activities of daily living and facilitate occupational performance. The AOTA states that these methods may be used as a precursor to activity or occupation. Administering PAMs as a treatment method without application to functional outcome or occupational performance is not considered occupational therapy, or sound practice.

Arguments against the use of physical agents in occupational therapy revolve around the contention that physical agents are not consistent with the basic philosophy of occupation, the hallmark being the use of purposeful activity, or occupation, to influence health and healing.[10] Others have contended that as occupational therapists, we have an ethical responsibility to use new technologies and interventions with our patients. These proponents have argued that the concept of occupational therapy to "diminish or correct pathology" places the onus of responsibility on the occupational therapist to utilize all mechanisms of intervention to facilitate occupational performance.[11] Failure to do so, in effect, would violate the Code of Ethics.

The issue and use of physical agents within the scope of practice for occupational therapy is, in fact, being forced by dramatic changes in health care and societal trends.

With the growth of managed care and its impetus to contain costs and limit health care expenditures, third party intermediaries and the federal government are less concerned with who provides what type of service, as long as it is safely, effectively, and appropriately provided. Additionally, the service must be consistent with appropriate standards of practice and service delivery, as well as being efficacious. The federal government, managed care organizations, and third party intermediaries are demanding that therapeutic interventions be related to and facilitate functional outcomes in our patients.

The challenge in today's dynamic health care environment is to treat our patients and clients with the most effective, yet low-cost technologies and interventions available, with the ultimate goal being improved occupational performance. By improving occupational performance, we facilitate the patient's ability to interact with his or her environment...perform occupations and roles of choice, and improve and enhance the individual's quality of life. Though other health professions which utilize physical agents in the treatment process espouse "function" and pay cursory attention to outcomes, the occupational therapist's unique perspective encompasses occupational performance issues at the level of the person-environment interaction, which is invaluable in selecting and utilizing physical agents in the treatment process.

Competency Issues

Aside from the philosophical issues inherent in physical agent modality use within the profession, the other primary argument relates to the issue of competency. One school of thought contends that the use of physical agent modalities is inconsistent with the basic philosophy of occupational therapy: that of purposeful activity, or occupation, to influence health and healing.[10-13] The use of occupation and purposeful activity is paramount to the profession, and as such, should not be abandoned. To this faction, physical agents do not address the basic human needs of independence in daily activities. To incorporate physical agents into our repertoire of treatment will open the profession to criticism, public confusion, political issues, and confrontation with physical therapy. This viewpoint, however, fails to address the issue that was articulated by Meyer,[14] who proposed in 1922 that occupation facilitates an individual's search for actuality, reality, a balance of time, and ultimately health. Physical agents can facilitate occupation by increasing the ability to function during activity through their influence on occupational performance components, eg, through pain reduction or tissue repair. Occupational therapists' strong background in psychosocial issues, activity analysis, and depth of understanding of occupation provide the therapist with a unique and valuable perspective on the use and application of physical agents. Research into many of the applications common for physical agents has demonstrated a relationship between outcomes and functional activity and improvement. Combining physical agents with occupation can improve the efficacy of many of the interventions and promote better outcomes.

Some therapists argue that physical agents are passive in nature, though therapists often use tools and techniques which allow the client to develop the ability to perform occupation or to prevent dysfunction, such as splinting and adaptive equipment. Others argue that the patients are engaged in active range of motion exercises during scar management, ultrasound, or whirlpool treatments, and if not, the interlude can be spent discussing occupational performance issues, collaborative goal setting, or patient education.[11] Rarely is the occupational therapist at a loss during this phase of narrative reasoning or interaction. The occupational therapist's ability to merge function and physical agents as part of the therapeutic intervention to ameliorate or compensate for deficits in occupational performance components is unique and valuable.

Competency is an issue which has been controversial within the profession and was one of the factors which led to the disagreement between the AOTA and the NBCOT. Competency, as it relates to physical agents, has also prevented occupational therapists from incorporating these agents and technologies into clinical practice. The AOTA has identified standards which require occupational therapy practitioners to receive specialized training for the proper use of physical agents. The AOTA contends that selection, application, and adjustment of physical agents is not entry-level practice, and requires continued training as the therapist's professional career evolves. Skill and training in physical agents can be achieved through fieldwork experience, on-the-job training, or post-professional education, such as continuing education, in-service training, or graduate education.[9] The AOTA also holds that practitioners have an ethical responsibility to possess basic information and the knowledge base, skills, or experience to safely and competently use physical agents. The AOTA contends that the theoretical background needed to use physical agents should include course work in anatomy and physiology; principles of chemistry and physics related to the properties of light, water, temperature, sound, and electricity; the physiological, neurophysiological, and electrophysiological changes that occur with the use of physical agents; and the response of normal and abnormal tissue to the agents. Course content should include information on pain control theories, wound healing principles, biophysical principles of thermal agents, and neurophysiologic mechanisms related to electrical stimulation.[6] The AOTA does concede that all practitioners should acquire an information base during entry-level education which defines physical agents, and hopefully grounds the use of physical agents within occupational therapy philosophy, standards, and ethics.

Unfortunately, the vast majority of occupational therapists who use physical agents learn on the job with little training occurring during higher-level education. In addition, there is a lack of competency testing, as well as any particular guidelines with regard to testing or frequency. There is little controversy among therapists about the necessity for training or education to acquire theoretical and technical competence with physical agents. Continuing education courses are currently considered the best method for gaining the skills necessary for deep thermal agents and those agents using the electromagnetic spectrum, such as neuromuscular electrical stimulation.[9] However, many therapists believe that physical agents should be considered part of entry-level occupational therapy programs and taught in the academic environment.[3,11] Though controversial, it would appear that the profession and educators move from their comfort area to assure that future therapists have the knowledge base and expertise to employ physical agents. As identified by the Intercommission Council, the challenge to the practitioner is not the acquisition of the technical skill in using physical agents, but in obtaining and developing the knowledge required to use physical agents as an adjunctive method with or in preparation for patient involvement in purposeful activity or occupation.

State Regulations

The AOTA contends that the use of physical agents is not entry-level practice and recommends additional post-professional education. Therapists should be cautious when utilizing a technology or technique which is "learned" from a manufacturer or sales representative during in-service training. Such continuing education often lacks the connection to, and the fundamental basics related to, the core concepts of occupation and function. Therapists utilizing physical agents within their clinical practice should have or obtain course work related to the principles of chemistry and physics associated with the properties of light, water, temperature, sound, and electricity. A thorough understanding of the wound healing process and the biophysiology related to the agents is necessary. Without continuing or professional level education and content, too many therapists apply physical agents without truly understanding or appreciating the benefits and efficacies of these technologies. Physical agents are often applied in a routine fashion without consideration of the type of injury, disability, or phase of healing, and the clinician may lack the clinical reasoning necessary to validly and effectively intervene using a physical agent.

Though the AOTA official position supports the use of physical agents in clinical practice, many states have established guidelines, restrictions, and licensing laws specific to physical agent use by occupational therapists. Therapists need to stay abreast of changes in local, state, and institutional rules and guidelines which may restrict or limit the use of physical agents by occupational therapists. States such as Florida, Georgia, Minnesota, and others specify training and competency standards for the use of physical agents by occupational therapists. Local, state, or institutional regulations and guidelines supercede the AOTA position statement on physical agents and therapists should research the regulations specific to their state and clinical practice.

Summary of States Requiring Competency in Physical Agents

The following states regulate the use of physical agents by occupational therapists and may define minimum competencies necessary to utilize physical agents by occupational therapists in clinical practice. Therapists should contact their respective state licensing and regulatory boards to obtain current information.

Florida

- Requires specific minimal competency level and training for the use of "electrical stimulation devices" and for "ultrasound device."
- Electrical stimulation requires education of at least 4 hours and performance of at least 5 treatments under supervision. Ultrasound requires didactic training of at least 4 hours and performance of at least 5 treatments under supervision.
- Continuing education can be obtained through educational programs, workshops, or seminars offered at a college or university approved for training by the AOTA, the American Physical Therapy Association (APTA), at clinical facilities affiliated with accredited colleges or universities, or through educational programs offered by the American Society of Hand Therapists (ASHT).[15]

Georgia

• Defines physical agent modalities as "...treatment techniques which utilize heat, light, sound, cold, electricity, or mechanical devices [and also means] electrical therapeutic modalities which induce heat or electrical current beneath the skin, including but not limited to therapeutic ultrasound, galvanism, microwave, diathermy, and electromuscular stimulation, and also means hydrotherapy."

• Requires 90 hours of instruction or training approved by the board.

• Specifies topics and subjects required for the 90 hours of instruction.

• No less than 36 contact hours must be directly related to the specific theories and practical application of physical agent modalities.

• Instruction or training shall include any activity relevant to the practice of physical agent modalities in occupational therapy and may include in-services education, conferences, workshops, seminars, and/or formal academic education.

• Documentation of proof of instruction or training must be submitted and may include official grade report or transcript to verify academic education.[16]

Kentucky

• Restricts the use of specific physical agent modalities as defined:"The practice of occupational therapy shall not include gait training; the use or application of electromodalities; accessory joint mobilizations; assessment of integrity and pathology of muscle, soft tissue and joint capsule; and postural or biomechanical analysis."

• Electromodalities are defined as "physical agents which supply or induce an electric current through the body, which make the body a part of the circuit."[17]

Massachusetts

• Defines treatment program to include "...the use of therapeutic agents or techniques in preparation for, or as an adjunct to, purposeful activity to enhance occupational performance."

• Defines occupational therapy as including "...utilizing designated modalities, superficial heat and cold, and neuromuscular facilitation techniques to improve or enhance joint motion or muscle function..."

• Requires "approaches taught in an occupational therapy curriculum, included in a program of professional education in occupational therapy, specific certification programs, continuing education or in-service education...must include documented educational goals and objective testing (written examination, practical examination, and/or written simulation or case study) to ascertain a level of competence."[18]

Minnesota

•Requires two levels of occupational therapy use with physical agent modalities:
    1. *Level 1*—use only under direct supervision
        a. Has received training in the theoretical properties of physical agent modalities
        b. Possesses written evidence of training or has achieved Certified Hand Therapist (CHT)
        c. Has completed clinical training through on-site demonstration
        d. Identifies specific criteria for physical agent modalities, electrical stimulation, and ultrasound
    2. *Level 2*—may use without supervision
        a. Requires 1800 hours in 2 years of employment in a clinical setting providing OT services
        b. Must meet one of the following:
            -Complete training in Level 1, develop treatment plan for six patients with the use of ice/cold, and 14 patients utilizing heat
            -Complete Level 1 training items using ice or heat with 20 patients in 1 year
            -Be certified as Certified Hand Therapist (CHT)
            -Demonstrates competency: electrical stimulation and ultrasound require the same competencies listed above for physical agents
            -Must complete 12 patients under supervision or must have completed CHT.[19]

Montana

•Includes employing PAMs as part of occupational therapy interventions; characterized as adjunctive methods used in conjunction with or in immediate preparation for patient involvement in purposeful activity.
•Defines physical agent modalities as "those modalities that produce a response in soft tissue through the use of light, water, temperature, sound, or electricity...superficial agents include hot packs, cold packs, ice, fluidotherapy, paraffin, water, and other commercially available superficial heating and cooling devices..." and restricts their use "to the shoulder, arm, elbow, forearm, wrist, and hand". Use of sound and electrical physical agent modality devices are also "limited to the elbow, forearm, wrist, and hand."
•Approval to use modalities (superficial agents) requires the unanimous approval of the licensing board committee.
•Must have documented completion of 16 contact hours of instruction or training within the nine criteria established by Regulation 37-24-105, MCA.
•Training may be obtained through educational programs, workshops or seminars offered at a college or university approved or recognized for training by the AOTA or the ASHT, or offered by clinical facilities affiliated with such a college or university, or by a licensed professional allowed to use the superficial modality. Professional must possess more than 1 year of clinical experience in the use of the superficial modality.

•Use of electrical or sound physical agents requires full approval of the licensing board and specifies instruction and training. May be an individual possessing CHT, and must complete 40 hours of instruction or training. The individual must document:

-15 contact hours of continuing education course work approved or recognized by the AOTA, ASHT, or by a licensed professional allowed to use deep modalities who has more than 1 year of clinical experience in the use of deep modalities and 100 treatments or 25 hours of instructor proctoring of sound and electrical physical agent modalities performed with patients

OR

-40 hours of direct instructor proctoring, which shall include at least 100 treatments.

•An individual lacking hand certification must complete 100 hours of instruction or training in sound and physical agent modalities. This must include 75 contact hours of continuing education course work approved or recognized by the AOTA or ASHT, and 100 treatments of sound and electrical physical agent modalities done on patients directly supervised by the instructor/proctor.

•Proctors must be preapproved by the board and show a certificate or proof of being a licensed professional allowed to use deep modalities with more than 1 year of clinical experience in the use of deep modalities, and in providing sound and electrical modalities.[20]

Nevada

•Allows the use of "physical therapeutic modalities and techniques which have been acquired through an appropriate program of education approved by the board...or through a program of continuing education or higher education."[21]

New York

•Allows for the use of "modalities and techniques based on approaches taught in an occupational therapy curriculum and included in a program of profession education in occupational therapy...and consistent with areas of individual competence."

•Treatment approaches are "based on, but not limited to, any one or more of the following...neurophysiological treatment approaches, muscle reeducation, superficial heat and cold..."[22]

North Dakota

•Defines modality as "the employment of or the method of employment of a therapeutic agent." Physical agent modalities are defined as "those modalities that produce a response in soft tissue through the use of light, water, temperature, sound, or electricity...and include but are not limited to paraffin baths, hot packs, cold packs, fluidotherapy, contrast baths, ultrasound, whirlpool, and electrical stimulation units."

•Specifies the educational background and scope of practice for the use of "specific procedures, activities, modalities, and techniques", as being displayed through "educational programs, including postprofessional programs, specific certification, in-service training, or professional experience approved by the board."

•Physical or therapeutic agents "...may be used only in preparation for, or as an adjunct to, purposeful activity to enhance occupational performance."

•Competency may "be obtained through accredited educational programs (including fieldwork education), specific certification, appropriate continuing education, in-service education, and postbaccalaureate higher education..."

•Continuing education specific to modalities and techniques must include "occupation as the common core of occupational therapy; must conform to the provisions of the North Dakota licensing board, and to the AOTA Code of Ethics and Standards of Practice."

•Specifies that occupational therapists, assistants, and students use modalities and techniques "only when the individual has received the theoretical and technical preparation necessary for safe and appropriate integration of the intervention in occupational therapy."[23]

Utah

•Defines occupational therapy services to include "applying physical agent modalities as an adjunct to or in preparation for purposeful activity..."

•Defines physical agent modalities as "specialized treatment procedures that produce a response in soft tissue through the use of light, water, temperature, sound, or electricity such as hotpacks, ice, paraffin, and electrical or sound currents."[24]

Therapists should always contact their licensing or regulatory boards at the state level to obtain current restrictions and/or guidelines related to physical agent use.

Summary

With the changes in health care and the evolution of occupational therapy delivery systems from the traditional inpatient, medical based practice model to one of community based, integrative models, occupational therapists are in a unique position to influence and expand their role in today's dynamic environment. Physical agents must not be considered a panacea, but an adjunct to facilitate an individual's occupational performance and integration into his or her community. Physical agents are additional tools and technologies which, when used appropriately, can facilitate the healing process. Occupational therapists have integrated new technologies and approaches in service delivery— augmentive technology, computers, state-of-the-art positioning and seating devices, dynamic splinting, environmental controls and technologies, work conditioning, and simulation. Clinicians and the profession must continue to embrace new technologies and interventions, while not discarding those concepts and tenets central to our profession. Many health professions see the value of our approach to the issues facing our patients, clients, and communities today and have attempted to incorporate our language into their service delivery. The government and third party intermediaries are also concerned about quality of life issues and the needs of the ill, elderly, and disabled to remain engaged within the environment. Managed care intermediaries and the federal government use terms such as ADL, self-care, disability, functional level, and independence in their expected outcomes.

As occupational therapists we must continue to remain visible, proactive, and dynamic. We must continue to explore and integrate new technologies and interventions consistent with our professional beliefs and scope of practice. Occupational therapy has a long history of continued evolution and change in response to societal and professional challenges. We must continue to evolve and adapt if we are to remain "a sufficiently vital and unique service for medicine to support and society to reward".[19] Failure to do so will create a vacuum quickly filled by another health profession.

References

1. American Occupational Therapy Association. *Physical Agent Modality Task Force Report*. Rockville, Md: 1991.

2. American Occupational Therapy Association. Official: AOTA statement on physical agent modalities. *AJOT*. 1991;45:1075.

3. Taylor E, Humphry R. Survey of physical agent modality use. *AJOT*. 1991;45:924-931.

4. Vogel K. Perceptions of practitioners, educators, and students concerning the role of the occupational therapy practitioner. *AJOT*. 1991;45:130-136.

5. Cornish-Painter C, Peterson C. Skill Acquisition and Competency Testing for Physical Agent Modality Use. *AJOT*. 1997;51:8.

6. American Occupational Therapy Association. *A Guide for the Preparation of Occupational Therapy Practitioners for the Use of Physical Agent Modalities*. Rockville, Md: 1994.

7. Glauner J, Ekes A, James A. A pilot study of the theoretical and technical competence and appropriate education for the use of nine physical agent modalities in occupational therapy practice. *AJOT*. 1997;51:9.

8. Funk DR. Occupational therapists' attitudes toward and use of physical agent modalities. *Journal of Occupational Therapy Students*. 1994;8:35-47.

9. American Occupational Therapy Association. Physical agent modalities position paper. *AJOT*. 1997;51:10.

10. West W, Weimer R. The issue is—Should the representative assembly have voted as it did, when it did, on occupational therapists' use of physical agent modalities? *AJOT*. 1991;45:1143-1147.

11. Ahlscwede K. The issue is—Views on physical agent modalities and specialization within occupational therapy: A rebuttal. *AJOT*. 1992;46:650-652.

12. West WL. A reaffirmed philosophy and practice of occupational therapy for the 1980s. *AJOT*. 1984;38:15-23.

13. McGuire MJ. AOTA releases draft position paper: Physical agent modalities. *OT Week*. 1991:6-7.

13. Fidler GS. Letters to the editor—Against use of physical agent modalities. *AJOT*. 1992;46;567.

14. Meyer A. The philosophy of occupation therapy. *Archives of Occupational Therapy*. 1922;1(1); 1-10.

15. Florida Board of Medicine, Occupational Therapy Practice Act, Florida State Licensure Law. 1991.

16. Georgia State Board of Occupational Therapy, Certificate of Validation for Use of Physical Agent Modalities. Rules of Georgia State Board of Occupational Therapy, Chapter 671-6, 1995.

17. Kentucky. Revised Statute, Chap.319A, Section 319A.010(2), Regulation 201 Kentucky Administrative Regulations 28;010A, Section 1.

18. Massachusetts Law. Chap. 667, Section 23A; Regulation: 259 CMR 3.00, 3.01 Definitions.

19. Minnesota Rules: 4666.0020 Definitions; 4666.0040; 4666.1000.

20. Montana Law. Title 37 Professions and Occupations, Chapter 24, Part I, Section 1. Definitions:(5) "Occupational Therapy"; Regulation: Rule 8, Chapter 35 Board of Occupational Therapists, Sub-Chapter 5 Use of Modalities.

21. Nevada Law: Chapter 383 Sec. 6. Definitions.

22. New York Regulation: N.Y. Title 8 Education, Section 76.7 (c)(3)(i)(ii), and (iii) Definition of occupational therapy practice: "treatment program".

23. North Dakota State Board of Occupational Therapy Practice. North Dakota Occupational Therapy Practice Handbook; 1993.

24. Utah Law: Title 58, Chapter 42a, Utah Code annotated; 58-42a-102. definitions; Regulation: Utah Administrative Code R156-42a-102 definitions.

25. Reilly M. Eleanor Clarke Slagle lecture: Occupational therapy can be one of the best ideas of 20th century medicine. *AJOT*. 1962;1:1-9.

Bibliography

American Occupational Therapy Association. Occupational therapist and modalities [Policy 1.23]. *AJOT*. 1983;37:816.

American Occupational Therapy Association. Registered occupational therapists and certified occupational therapy assistants and modalities [Policy 1.25]. *AJOT*. 1991;45:1112-1113.

American Occupational Therapy Association. Position paper: Physical agent modalities. *AJOT*. 1992;46:1090-1091.

American Occupational Therapy Association. Use of adjunctive modalities in occupational therapy. *AJOT*. 1992;46:1075-1081.

American Occupational Therapy Association. *Occupational Therapy Code of Ethics*. Rockville, Md: 1994.

American Occupational Therapy Association. Standards of practice for occupational therapy. *AJOT*. 1994;48:1039-1043.

American Occupational Therapy Association. *States Regulating Physical Agent Modalities*. Bethesda, Md:1996.

American Physical Therapy Association. Section on clinical electrophysiology's curriculum content guidelines for physical agents and electrotherapy. Alexandria, Va: 1995.

Bailey D, Schwartzberg S. *Ethical and Legal Dilemmas in Occupational Therapy*. Philadelphia, Pa: F.A. Davis; 1995.

Baum C, Law M. Occupational therapy practice: focusing on occupational performance. *AJOT*. 1997;51:277-288.

Commission on Education Physical Agent Modalities Task Force. Educational preparation for use of physical agent modalities in occupational therapy [Report]. AOTA. Rockville, Md: 1993.

English C, Kasch M, Silverman P, Walker S. The issue is--On the role of the occupational therapist in physical disabilities. *AJOT*. 1982;36:199-202.

Michigan Hand SIS, Physical Agents/Modalities, (1997), Unpublished.

Pedretti LW. *Therapeutic Modalities: Occupational Therapy Practice Skills for Physical Dysfunction,*

4th ed. St. Louis, Mo: Mosby; 1996:300-312.

Pedretti LW, Smith RO, McGuire MJ. Use of adjunctive modalities in occupational therapy. *AJOT*. 46(12):1075-81.

Reynolds C. OTs and PAMs: A physical therapist's perspective. *OT Week*. September 1994;17.

Rose H. Physical agent modalities: OT's contribution. *OT Week*. September 1994;17.

Trombly CA. Include exercise in "purposeful activity" [Letter to the editor]. *AJOT*. 1982;36:467-468.

Vogel KA. Perception of practitioners, educators, and students concerning the role of the occupational therapy practitioner. *AJOT*. 1991;45:130-136.

West W. Nationally speaking—Perspectives on the past and future, Part 1. *AJOT*. 1989;44:787.

Chapter Two

Wound Healing

Learning Objectives

1. Identify the phases of wound healing.
2. Describe the anatomy of the skin.
3. List the classification systems describing pressure ulcers and wounds.
4. Identify the factors which influence or impair the healing process.
5. Discuss the clinical decision-making in assessing wounds and wound healing.

Terminology

Approximation	Keloid
Dermis	Partial-thickness
Epidermis	Picture frame
Epithelialization	Proliferation
Fibroblasts	Purulent
Full-thickness	Remodeling
Granulation tissue	Serosanguanous
Hypertrophic scar	Serous
Inflammation	Wound classification

An understanding of the wound healing process and an appreciation of the sequence of events which occurs following injury are necessary to be able to determine appropriate interventions and technologies which may facilitate healing and positively influence the process. Wound healing is a complex process involving myriad events and is influenced by both physical and psychological components. Initial insult or injury to the body causes a series of physiologic responses which are overlapping and sequenced, ultimately resulting in normal healing. Influencing wound healing is dependent upon the therapist understanding the process of repair and the factors which affect the repair process, and then clinically reasoning through the interventions and technologies that may impact the outcome.

Skin Anatomy

The skin is composed of two primary layers, the epidermis and the dermis. The skin is the largest organ of the body and functions as a barrier between the body and the external environment. The epidermis is approximately 0.04 mm thick, and the dermis is approximately 0.5 mm thick. The epidermis is the outer epithelial layer which provides a protective barrier to injury, contamination, and light. The epidermis is avascular and also functions to prevent dehydration of the underlying tissues.

The dermis is vascularized and composed of collagen and elastin fibrous connective tissues which give the skin its strength and resilience. The vascular supply of the dermis also nourishes the epidermis and is responsible, in part, for regulating body temperature. Hair follicles, sebaceous and sweat glands are located in the dermis and help to provide the secretions which lubricate and keep the skin soft and flexible. Nerve endings are also located in the dermis, along with the receptors for pain, touch, heat, and cold. Subcutaneous layers consisting of fat tissues and connective tissues are located below the dermis. These subcutaneous layers protect the underlying tissue and provide insulation, support, and cushioning to withstand pressure and stress.

Wound Classification

There are a number of wound classification systems used to describe the etiology and severity of a wound. The most common classifications used by therapists are based on the tissue layers and depth of tissue destruction, the National Pressure Ulcer Advisory Panel (NPUAP)[1], and on wound color, such as the Marion Laboratories red/yellow/black color system.[2,3]

Pressure Ulcers: Four Stage System

The NPUAP pressure ulcer staging system is most frequently used to classify ulcers. It is recommended for use with wounds caused by pressure or tissue perfusion such as diabetic neuropathic ulcers. [4] The NPUAP classification uses a four stage system which describes pressure ulcers by anatomic depth and the soft tissue layers which are involved. Pressure ulcers are often referred to as bedsores, decubitus ulcers, or pressure

The Four Stage System for Pressure Ulcers

Stage I: Nonblanchable erythema of intact skin; the presaging lesion of skin ulceration. Discoloration of the skin, warmth, edema, induration, or hardness may also be indicators.

Stage II: Partial-thickness skin loss involving epidermis and/or dermis. The ulcer is superficial and presents clinically as an abrasion, a blister, or a shallow crater.

Stage III: Full-thickness skin loss involving damage or necrosis of subcutaneous tissue which may extend down to, but not through, underlying fascia. The ulcer presents clinically as a deep crater with or without undermining of adjacent tissue.

Stage IV: Full-thickness skin loss with extensive destruction, tissue necrosis or damage to muscle, bone, or supporting structures (eg, tendon, joint capsule).[2]

sores. Pressure ulcers are caused by localized areas of tissue necrosis, which are often associated with compression between a bony prominence and an external surface for an extended period of time. The four stage system is commonly used to describe wound severity and to establish treatment protocols and interventions.[5]

A primary difficulty inherent in the stage system of wound classification is that identification of the wound cannot be done if the area is covered by eschar or necrotic tissue until it is removed. Staging of the wound should be used only as a diagnostic tool to describe the severity of the wound, not the healing of the wound.[6]

Depth of Tissue Involvement

Wounds can also be classified according to the depth of the tissue involved, and the thickness of the skin loss—partial- or full-thickness. This classification system is most often used for skin tears, donor sites, surgical wounds, and burns. Partial-thickness wounds involve the epidermal layer and may include the superficial layer of the dermis. Partial-thickness wounds do not extend through the dermis, the second layer of the skin. Partial-thickness wounds heal by regeneration, known as epithelialization, and may be characterized by a crust or covering consisting of blood and debris particles. Because of their superficial nature, partial-thickness wounds heal faster than full-thickness wounds. Partial-thickness wounds are shallow, moist and may be painful due to the loss of the epidermal coverings with exposure of the nerve endings. The wound base often appears as bright pink-red.

By contrast, full-thickness wounds involve the epidermis, dermis, and subcutaneous tissues. Subcutaneous tissue wounds may extend into muscles, fascia, tendons, and bone, depending on the depth of injury. Full-thickness wounds may involve necrotic tissue or infection. Full-thickness wound healing is a complex process often referred to as secondary intention healing. This process consists of three phases of inflammatory, proliferative, and remodeling. These phases of the healing process are not singular events and may overlap. Full-thickness wounds heal by secondary intention, which involves fibroplasia or the formation of granulation tissue with contraction of the wound. [7,8]

Red/Yellow/Black Wound Classification

Wounds which are classified according to their surface color are described using the three-color concept of red, yellow, or black. This system is frequently used in the clinic due to its simplicity. Red wounds are clean, healing, and granulating appropriately without complications. The goal is to provide a moist wound environment and minimize any damage to the newly formed tissue. Yellow wounds may indicate the possibility of infection and the need for debridement and cleaning of the area. Yellow may also indicate the presence of necrotic tissue. The yellow tissue contains devitalized slough, or fibrous exudate which can promote bacterial growth and infection. The goal of treatment at this stage is to remove the exudate and debris. Black wounds indicate the presence of necrotic or dead tissue which provides a medium for bacterial growth and proliferation. A black wound requires cleaning and debridement of the area and is often encountered with full-thickness leg/foot ulcers, and in patients with gangrene or deep burns. Rarely are wounds exclusively one color, and most manifest all three colors depending on the amount of necrotic tissue as well as systemic and local influences on the healing process.

Wound Closure

Healthy wounds follow a logical progression of healing in a timely fashion. However, external factors such as trauma or compromised systems may cause complications and negatively affect the healing process. There are three types of surgical wound healing: primary closure, secondary closure, and delayed primary closure.

Primary or "intention" closure refers to wounds which occur when full-thickness surgical incisions or acute wound edges are approximated and sutured together. Primary closure is most often used when there is minimal skin loss and the acute wound edges can be approximated or apposed and aligned together. Secondary closure is used on wounds which are open, large, and full-thickness. Secondary wounds are left open following surgery and display soft tissue loss. The healing process with secondary wounds takes longer because the area is allowed to heal by production of connective tissue (scar). Delayed primary closure, or tertiary intention, occurs when the wound is initially left open for a short period of time followed by approximation and closure of the wound. Delayed primary closure most often occurs in complex wounds which may be contaminated or may develop infection during the acute phase of the healing process. [9,10]

In general, the normal healing process in a surgical wound should take approximately 4 weeks, at which point the area should display granular tissue and be covered with epithelial tissue. The wound healing process and rate of healing can be affected by the patient's age, underlying and associated systemic conditions, nutritional status, tissue perfusion, and vascularity. Infections within the wound also affect the healing process negatively, slowing collagen production. Dry wounds are at a disadvantage with regard to the rate of healing. Moist wounds heal at a quicker rate, as the moist environment facilitates epithelialization and reduces crust or scab formation. Epidermal

Table 2-1. Local and Systemic Indices of Inflammation	
Local Signs	**Systemic Signs**
Redness	Fever
Swelling	Leukocytosis
Heat	
Pain	

cells require a moist surface to migrate across the wound surface. There are a wide variety of dressings which can facilitate the healing process and the reader is encouraged to explore the options available.[12-16]

Phases of Normal Wound Healing

In a "normal" or healthy individual, the body's response to an injury is well ordered and sequenced, though the stages of repair may overlap. The healing process has been described as having either three or four phases, based on whether epithelialization is viewed as a distinct phase of repair or is included under the phase of proliferation.[17-20]

Phase I: Inflammatory

The inflammatory phase of healing is the body's initial response to an injury. Clotting and vasoconstriction (hemostasis) occur at the initial time of injury and decrease blood loss. The inflammatory response is both vascular and cellular and is the body's response to rid itself of bacteria, foreign matter, and dead tissue. The inflammatory response occurs quickly, and is associated with changes in skin color (red, blue, purple), temperature (heat), turgor (swelling), and sensation (pain), and may include a loss of function. Acute inflammation begins immediately at the time of the injury. The acute inflammatory phase usually lasts for 24-48 hours and is completed within 7 days, though a subacute phase of inflammation may continue for approximately 2 weeks (Table 2-1). [21]

The initial response to an injury is characterized by vascular changes at the site of injury. Vasoconstriction occurs with platelet aggregation along the endothelium of the injured blood vessel. These platelets release vasoconstrictive, chemotactic and growth-promoting substances which facilitate the formation of fibrin clots, preventing excessive hemorrhage. The release of vasoactive substances, such as histamine and prostaglandins, as well as stimulation of local sensory nerve endings, causes a local reflex action leading to vasodilation and increased permeability.[22] This produces vasocongestion and leakage of the serous fluid into the wound bed, causing the wound to become erythematous, edematous, and warm with exudate (Figure 2-1). Vasodilation and leakage into the wound area continues for several days. Leukocytes or white blood cells (WBC) also migrate to the area. Neutrophils migrate through the blood vessel walls to phagocytose bacteria and other foreign contaminants. Leukocyte migration occurs within 20 minutes after the initial insult.

Figure 2-1. Inflammation process. A. Tissue injury. B. (Cross section) vasodilation of arterioles. Result: heat/redness. C. Capillaries leak fluid (exudate). Result: pain and swelling. Illustration by Kim Bartlett. Used with permission.

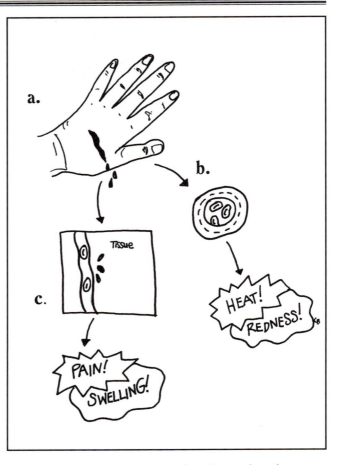

Monocytes are converted into macrophages entering the tissue by day two. Macrophages are critical for wound healing and engulf the bacteria and debris, cleaning the wound and breaking down necrotic tissue. Macrophages play an important role in the healing process—secreting growth factors, and mediating the formation of blood vessels via angiogenesis. Chemical changes in the tissue are due in part to the histamine released by the mast cells and the prostaglandin which is released by the injured cell membrane.[23] The blood serum contains proteolytic enzymes which degrade necrotic tissue at the wound site and assist in cleaning the wound bed, further facilitating the healing process (Figure 2-2). The process of inflammation is vital to the healing process and a balance must be achieved to ensure appropriate and timely healing (Table 2-2).

Phase 2: Proliferative

The proliferative phase of recovery has a number of different titles, including fibroplastic phase, granulation, and epithelialization phase. In the proliferative phase of healing, the area of damage is filled with new connective tissue and the wound is covered with new epithelium. The primary components of this phase of healing are granulation, epithelialization, and wound contraction. This process overlaps the inflammatory phase, continuing until the wound is healed. Epithelialization occurs through a series of events, including mobilization, migration, proliferation and differentiation. Wound contraction is also occurring with red granulation tissue forming, which consists of newly formed

Table 2-2.
Sequence of the Inflammatory Response

Vasodilation occurs in response to tissue injury

Tissues become red and warm

Capillary permeability increases

Exudate flows into the injured tissues
Tissues become swollen
Blood clot forms

Leukocytes accumulate at the injury site (Leukocytosis)

Phagocytosis occurs

Cellular repair begins

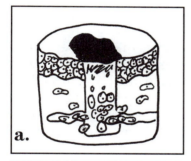

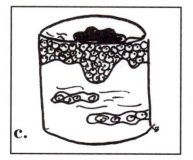

Figure 2-2. Proliferation. A. Epidermis. B. Scab, regenerating epithelium, granulation tissue ingrowth, capillary budding. C. Regenerated epithelium, fibrosis complete. Illustrations by Kim Bartlett. Used with permission.

a.

b.

c.

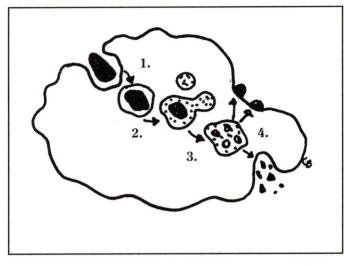

Figure 2-3. Macrophage during Phagocytosis. 1. Macrophage engulfs particle. 2. Phagocytic vesicle fuses with lysosome to form phagolysosome. 3. Antigen in phagolysosome is partially degraded and portions are re-expressed on surface. 4. Waste expelled by exocytosis. Illustra-tion by Kim Bartlett. Used with permission.

collagen and blood vessels. [24] Granulation tissue fills in the wound site. Wound contraction decreases the size of the affected area and begins approximately 5 days after the injury, peaking at approximately 2 weeks.

The process of wound contraction closes the wound, resulting in a smaller area requiring repair by scar formation. Wound contraction should be complete by approximately 2 to 3 weeks after the injury. Wound contraction occurs through the action of myofibroblasts (Figure 2-3). Range of motion exercises and functional activities assist in controlling contraction and ensure that the surrounding skin is supple and mobile. Myofibroblasts connect to the wound margins, pulling the epidermal layer inward and producing the characteristic picture frame beneath the skin. [25] The shape of the picture frame predicts the speed of contraction, with linear wounds contracting rapidly, square or rectangular wounds contracting at a moderate pace, and circular wounds being the slowest to close and contract.

Fibroblasts are the cells which are responsible for fibroplasia and are stimulated by lactic acid, ascorbic acid, and other cofactors which stimulate the fibroblasts to synthesize collagen. Cross-linkage of the collagen tissue provides the wound with its tensile strength and durability. The tensile strength of remodeled skin is weaker and will never exceed 75-80%. [26]

Cellular activity in the second phase of repair consists of macrophage-stimulated collagen synthesis, formation of a network of blood capillaries, wound contraction, and wound epithelialization. The second phase of healing is completed when epithelialization has resurfaced the wound, a collagen layer has been formed, and initial remodeling is complete.

Phase 3: Remodeling

The remodeling phase of wound healing has also been termed the maturation phase. The remodeling phase occurs approximately 2 weeks after the injury and may continue for up to a year or longer. The remodeling phase is characterized by a relative balance of collagen synthesis and collagen lysis, the formation and breakdown of collagen. The scar which was formed during fibroplasia is dense and disorganized. During remodeling, the scar may appear "rosier" than normal and is indicative that remodeling is occurring. This phase of remodeling normally provides the scar with its maximum tensile strength as well as changes in its appearance. [27]

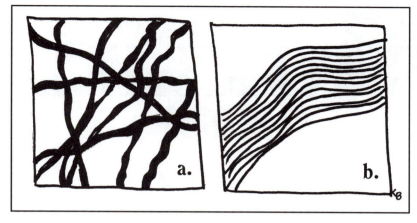

Figure 2-4. A. Collagen; new wound randomly laid. B. Normal dermis. Illustration by Kim Bartlett. Used with permission.

Scar tissue consists of disorganized collagen fibers laid down by the fibroblasts, is randomly arranged, and different from the surrounding tissue (Figure 2-4). As the wound matures during remodeling, collagen lysis increases and the scar becomes more elastic, smoother, and the fibers stronger. If collagen synthesis exceeds collagen lysis, hypertrophic scarring or keloid formation may occur. Keloid scars extend beyond the boundary of the wound and appear raised. Hypertrophic scars occur within the area of the wound and may eventually decrease in size and shape.[28] One mechanism frequently used to control the development of hypertrophic or keloid scarring is the application of pressure garments. Wearing of the pressure garments is continued until the process of remodeling is complete.

As the process of remodeling continues, the collagen fibers are randomly oriented and arranged in a linear and lateral orientation. As the scar continues to mature and the process of collagen synthesis and lysis continues, these fibers assume some of the characteristics of the tissue they are replacing. There are two primary theories which explain how collagen fibers become aligned: induction theory and tension theory. [29] Induction theory proposes that the scar tissue attempts to mimic the characteristics of the tissue it is healing. Tension theory purports that internal and external stresses which are placed on the wound affect and align the fibers during remodeling. Tension theory is supported, to an extent, by several studies suggesting that adding tension during healing increases the tensile strength of soft tissue structures and bone, whereas immobilizing the area produces a loss of tensile strength and collagen fiber organization.[30] Tension theory, in part, accounts for the use of dynamic splinting, serial casting, continuous passive motion (CPM) devices, positional stretching, neuromuscular electrical stimulation (NMES), and the use of silastic gel pads and compression garments in the treatment process (Table 2-3).[31]

Factors Impacting Wound Healing

As remodeling continues, the bright pink color of the immature scar softens, flattens and becomes white and soft. Full maturity for a scar may continue for up to 2 years. There are, however, a number of factors which may affect the rate and outcome of normal healing. External and internal factors may delay or impair the healing process during any of the three phases of healing, and a balance is required to ensure appropriate healing. The presence of foreign objects or microorganisms also impair the healing process. Common microorganisms which cause infections in wounds include

Table 2-3.
Normal Wound Healing and Repair: Sequence of Events

24 Hours After Injury:

  Epithelialization begins
  Cell regeneration

3-5 Days After Injury:

  Fibroplasia occurs
  Neovascularization occurs
  Granulation tissue forms

2-4 Weeks After Injury:

  Wound remodeling begins
  Collagen gathers into large fibers
  Scar formation

Pseudomonas eruginosa and *Staphylococcus aureus.* Clinical signs of an infected wound include increased erythema, heat, edema, pus, increased body temperature, pain, purulent drainage, and an uncharacteristic odor. The risk of infection can be minimized through proper debridement procedures, cleaning, and dressing techniques. The presence of foreign bodies, necrotic tissue, and eschar also impairs the healing of the wound and may predispose the wound to bacterial infection. Surgical debridement of the eschar, necrotic tissue, or debris may minimize the adverse effects the foreign material may have on healing.

Nutrition also plays a key role in the healing process, and a deficiency in any nutrient, vitamins A, C, and E, or trace metals such as zinc or copper, may impact the healing process.[32] Systemic diseases such as diabetes mellitus, atherosclerosis, acquired immune deficiency syndrome (AIDS), and other vascular diseases may also have a pronounced adverse effect on wound healing. Diabetes mellitus is a major cause of poor wound healing. Patients with poorly controlled diabetes have slower rates of healing, due in part to decreased circulation secondary to atherosclerosis, and diabetic neuropathy which decreases sensation in the extremities, particularly the lower extremity, which may lead to ulcerations at pressure points with weight-bearing. Patients using systemic medications such as steroids, nonsteroidal antiinflammatory drugs (NSAIDS), chemotherapeutic agents, antibiotics, and anticoagulants will impact the normal healing process.[33] The aging process and associated physiological changes which occur in the elderly slow the healing response. Delayed granulation and a decreased inflammatory response is more common in the elderly, along with a slow rate of epithelialization and a decreased tensile strength (Table 2-4).[34]

Table 2-4.
Factors Affecting Healing and Repair

Systemic Factors:

> Nutrition
> Hematologic abnormalities
> Diabetes mellitus
> Antimetabolite, immunosuppressive, radiation therapy
> Age

Local Factors:

> Infection
> Adequacy of blood supply
> Foreign bodies

Documentation

The involvement of the therapist in the management of open wounds and wound healing will depend on the clinical site, experience of the therapist, and involvement of other medical staff, such as nursing. Occupational therapists are often involved in the management of sprains, strains, and acute injuries, and those practicing in orthopedics may be more deeply involved in the management of wounds and the healing process. It is beyond the scope of this text to describe the wide variety and application of the types of dressings available. Therapists should be well versed in the indications and contraindications of each type of dressing, from gauze to hydrocolloids. Therapists requiring further information on dressings should review the number of excellent texts available on the subject.

The primary purpose of wound assessment is to obtain baseline information on what the wound looks like prior to treatment intervention. Additionally, clear and appropriate documentation demonstrates the effectiveness of the interventions to third party payers. The therapist should use a systematic approach when managing wounds. Questions such as: What caused the wound? Was it due to pressure, laceration, thermal (heat) or nonthermal (cold), chemical, or caused by a vascular impairment or disease process? Is the wound bleeding? (Review the medical record for the platelet count and to assist in determining clotting efficiency or if the patient is taking any medications such as coumadin or heparin which may impede clotting.) What is the extent and depth of the wound; is it superficial, partial- or full-thickness, does it involve muscle, tendon, or bone? Is there foreign debris or dead necrotic tissue present? The presence of eschars may impede the healing process and facilitate wound infection. Does the wound show signs of a clinical infection? Are there clinical signs such as increased erythema, edema, purulence, body temperature, pain, changes in the color of the exudate, or an uncharacteristic or foul odor? Clinicians should review any lab work for confirmation on cultures which may have been taken or for increased white blood cell count which may account for infections.

When documenting a wound assessment, the therapist should include the following information:
- Anatomical location and area of the wound
- Size of the wound (length, width, depth)
- Shape of the wound: draw the shape or use one of the many documentation patterns available
- Presence of dead or necrotic tissue and its color (black, brown, yellow)
- Description of the wound exudate (purulent pus, milky), serous (clean, yellowish), serosanguanous (pinkish)
- Presence of any healthy granulation tissue at the base or epithelialization at the wound margins
- Description of the surrounding intact skin: presence of erythema, heat, pain, edema

Determining an appropriate diagnosis and intervention occurs following the evaluation of the problem. The patient's potential prognosis and level of improvement is determined and aids in identifying appropriate interventions and technologies which will help achieve the stated goals.[35]

Physical agent technologies have been demonstrated to be effective in influencing and impacting the healing process. In patients with open wounds, the use of hydrotherapy to cleanse and debride the wound may be effective. Electrical stimulation has been shown to assist in debridement as well as to facilitate epithelialization and contraction of the wound. Ultrasound has been used to promote wound healing during the proliferative and remodeling phases, and is used extensively in the management of soft tissue inflammation. [36-38] The use of continuous passive movement devices to assist with scar management and to promote healing is well documented, as is the use of early controlled mobilization through the application of dynamic splints.[39,40]

Summary

The wound healing process has been described as an overlapping cascade of events which include the three primary phases of inflammation, proliferation, and remodeling. An understanding of the healing process and the stages of recovery are vital for the therapist to aid in determining functional outcomes and to be able to influence the healing process through the potential application of physical agent technologies and interventions. Identifying an appropriate intervention and treatment plan to manage the wound and injury through debridement, facilitating healing through physical technologies, selection of appropriate dressings, and engaging an individual in developmentally and occupationally appropriate activities are all critical to facilitating an individual's return to normal occupational roles and performance.

Case Study

MJ is a 77 y/o female referred to occupational therapy following a fall which occurred at home in the early spring. Though there were no fractures, MJ fell, striking her face and landing on her right hand, rolling onto the extremity. MJ is an active woman who lives alone, enjoys gardening and canning the fruits of her labor in the fall.

She is concerned over her inability to fully flex or extend the digits of her right hand and the stiffness which has developed in her wrist. Clinical evaluation reveals an alert, social female, in no apparent distress. Primary complaint is of "stiffness and aching" in her right hand and wrist. Examination reveals edema and discoloration over the entire dorsal aspect of the hand. The skin is taut, with a purplish-blue color indicating a large hematoma. The right side of the patient's face also displays a large, dark purple-blue hematoma with areas of yellow. There is no drainage noted, but the extent of the hematoma and the associated edema are limiting the patient's active movement and prehension patterns. MJ relates that she is able to dress herself and take care of her basic ADL needs, but is having difficulty with fastenings, manipulating objects using the right hand, higher level homemaking tasks such as cleaning, and activities requiring bilateral use of the hands.

Further evaluation of the patient included grip/pinch strength, prehension patterns, object manipulation, sensation, ADL components and measurements, determination of social support systems, and her adjustment to the injury. The treatment plan was established and included hydrotherapy to warm the tissue and increase bloodflow, and for its cellular effects. During the whirlpool treatment, MJ was encouraged to perform gentle exercises for muscle pumping and strengthening and to prevent edema in the dependent position. Following whirlpool, treatment using ultrasound was added to promote absorption of the hematoma. Because of the depth of the tissue involvement and size of the area, the hematoma took approximately 2 weeks to resolve. The treatment protocol for the ultrasound was 3 MHz, 0.5 W/cm2, pulsed at 20% duty cycle for 6 minutes. A frequency of 3 MHz was selected due to the hematoma's location on the dorsal aspect of the hand and wrist, a superficial area. The nonthermal effects of the ultrasound were used to facilitate the biologic process of repair through its cellular effect of stable cavitation and/or acoustic streaming. Occupational activities proceeded the physical agents, with MJ engaging in a variety of activities facilitating active prehension patterns and use of the right hand and wrist.

References

1. Van Rijswijk L. Frequency of reassessment of pressure ulcers, NPUAP Proceedings. *Adv Wound Care.* July/August 1995;8(4 Supp):19-24.

2. National Pressure Ulcer Advisory Panel (NPUAP). Pressure ulcers: prevalence, cost and risk assessment: Consensus development conference statement. *Decubitus.* 1989;292:24-28.

3. Wagner FW. The dysvascular foot: A system for diagnosis and treatment. *Foot Ankle.* 1981;3:64-122.

4. Bergstrom N. *Treatment of Pressure Ulcers.* Clinical Practice Guideline No. 15. AHCPR Publication N. 95-0652. Rockville, MD: Agency for Health Care Policy and Research, U.S. Department of Health and Human Services; December 1994.

5. Shea JD. Pressure sore: classification and management. *Clin Orthop.* 1975;112:89-100.

6. Krasner D, Weir D. Recommendations for using reverse staging to complete the M.D.S.-2. *Ostomy Wound Manage.* 1997;43(3):14-17.

7. Hess CT. *Nurse's Clinical Guide, Wound Care.* Springhouse, PA: Springhouse; 1995.

8. Nemeth AJ, Eaglstein WH, Taylor JR, Peerson LJ, Falanga V. Faster healing and less pain in skin biopsy sites treated with an occlusive dressing. *Arch Derm.* 1991;127:1679-1683.

9. Walters MD, Dombroski RA, Davidson SA, Mandel PC, Gibbs RS. Reclosure of disrupted abdominal incisions. *Obstet Gynecol.* 1990;76:597-602.

10. Herman GC, Bagi P, Christofferson I. Early secondary suture versus healing by second intention of incisional abscesses. *Surg Gynecol Obstet.* 1988;167:16-18.

11. Dodson MK, Magann EF, Meeks GR. A randomized comparison of secondary closure and secondary intention in patients with superficial wound dehiscence. *Obstet Gynecol*. 1992;80:321-324.

12. Rohrich RJ, Pittman CE. A clinical comparison of DuoDERM CGF and OpSite donor site dressings. *Wounds*. 1991;3:221-226.

13. Hermans MHE, Van Wingerden S. Treatment of industrial wounds with DuoDERM bordered: a report on medical and patient comfort aspects. *J Soc Occup Med*. 1990;40:101-102.

14. Poulsen TD, Freund KG. Polyurethane film (OpSite) vs. impregnated gauze (jelonet) in the treatment of outpatient burns: a prospective, randomized study. *Burns*. 1991;17:59-61.

15. Phillips TJ, Kapoor V, Provan A, Ellerin T. A randomized prospective study of a hydroactive dressing vs. conventional treatment after shave biopsy excision. *Arch Derm*. 1993;129:859-860.

16. Bolton L, Van Rijswijk L. Wound dressings: meeting clinical and biological needs. *Derm Nurs*. 1991;3:146-161.

17. Cooper D. The physiology of wound healing: an overview. In: *Chronic Wound Care*. Wayne, PA: Health Management Publications; 1990:1-11.

18. Reed B, Zarro V. Inflammation and repair and the use of thermal agents. In: Michlovitz SL. *Thermal Agents in Rehabilitation*. 2nd ed. Philadelphia, Pa: F.A. Davis; 1990:3.

19. Kloth LC, McCulloch JM. The inflammatory response to wounding. In: McCulloch JM, Kloth LC, Feedar JA, eds. *Wound Healing: Alternatives in Management*. 2nd ed. Philadelphia, Pa: FA Davis; 1995:3.

20. Hunt TK, Hussain M. Can wound healing be a paradigm for tissue repair? *Med Sci Sports Exerc*. 1994;26:755-758.

21. Harding KG. Wound care: putting theory into clinical practice. In: Krasner D, ed. *Chronic Wound Care: A Clinical Source Book for Health Care Professionals*. 1st ed. Wayne, PA: Health Management Publications;1990:24.

22. Bryant WM. Wound healing. *Clin Symp*. 1977;29:1-36.

23. Hardy MA. The biology of scar formation. *Phys Ther*. 1989;69:1014.

24. Messer MS. Wound care. *Crit Care Nurs Q*. 1989;11:17.

25. Hardy MA. The biology of scar formation. *Phys Ther*. 1989;69:1014-1023.

26. Schumann D. The nature of wound healing. *AORN J*. 1982;35:1067-1077.

27. Hardy MA. The biology of scar formation. *Phys Ther*.1989;69:1014-1032.

28. Peacock EE, Madden JW, Trier WC. Biologic basis for the treatment of keloids and hypertrophic scars. *South Med J*. 1970;63:755-760.

29. Gogia P. *Clinical Wound Management*. Thorofare, NJ: SLACK Incorporated; 1995:7.

30. Arem AJ, Madden JW. Effects of stress on healing wounds. I. Intermittent noncyclical tension. *J Surg Res*. 1976;20:93-102.

31. Sussman C, Bates-Jensen B. *Wound Care*. Gaithersburg, MD: Aspen Publishers; 1998:40.

32. Pollack SV. Wound healing: a review. III. Nutritional factors affecting wound healing. *J Dermatol Surg Oncol*. 1979;5:615-619.

33. Hunt TK. Disorders of wound healing. *World J Surg*. 1980;4:271-277.

34. Mulder G, Brazinsky BA, Seeley J. Factors complicating wound repair. In: McCulloch JM, Kloth LC, Feeder JA, eds. *Healing Alternatives in Management*. 2nd ed. Philadelphia, Pa: F.A. Davis; 1995;47-59.

35. Doenges MD, Moorhouse MF, Burley JT. *Application of Nursing Process and Nursing Diagnosis*. 2nd ed. Philadelphia, Pa: F.A. Davis; 1995.

36. Unger P, Eddy J, Raimastry S. A controlled study of the effect of high voltage pulsed current (HVPC) on wound healing. *Phys Ther*. 1991;71(suppl): S119.

37. Unger PC. A randomized clinical trial of the effect of HVPC on wound healing. *Phys Ther*. 1991;71(suppl): S118.

38. Kalinowski DP, Brogan MS, Sleeper MD. A practical technique for disinfecting electrical stimulation apparatuses used in wound treatment. *Phys Ther*. 1996;12:1340-1347.

39. Woo SL, Gelberman RH, Cobb NG, et al. The importance of controlled passive mobilization on flexor tendon healing: A biochemical study. *Acta Orthop Scand*. 1981;52:615.

40. Gelberman RH, Woo SL, Lothringer K, et al. Effects of early intermittent passive immobilization on healing canine flexor tendons. *J Hand Surg*. 1982;7:170.

Bibliography

Dabrowski R, Masinski C, Olczak A. The role of histamine in wound healing: the effect of high doses of histamine on collagen and glycosaminoglycan in wounds. *Agents Actions*. 1997;7:210-224.

Kincaid C, Lavoie K. Inhibition of bacterial growth in vitro following stimulation with high voltage, monophasic pulsed current. *Phys Ther*. 1990;70:20-33.

Kloth LC. Electrical stimulation in tissue repair. In: McColloch JM, Kloth LC, Feeder JA, eds. *Wound Healing Alternatives in Management*. 2nd ed. Philadelphia PA: F.A. Davis;1995:202.

McDiarmid T, Burns P. Clinical applications of therapeutic ultrasound. *Physiother J Chartered Soc Physiotherapy*. 1097;73(4):14-21.

Myers JA. Wound healing and the use of modern surgical dressing. *Pharm J*. 1982;220:103-104.

Sussman C. *Ultrasound for Wound Healing*. Monograph. Houston, TX: The Chattanooga Group;1993.

Swanson G. Functional outcome report: the next generation in physical therapy reporting. In: Stewart D, Ablen S, eds. *Documenting Physical Therapy Outcomes*. St. Louis, MO: Mosby Year Book; 1993:101-134.

Weiss DS. Pulsed electrical stimulation decreases scar thickness at split-thickness graft donor sites. *J Invest Dermatol*. 1989;92:530.

Whiston RJ. Application of high frequency ultrasound to the objective assessment of healing wounds. In: *Proceedings of the 2nd Conference on Advances in Wound Management*. London: Macmillan Press;1992:26-29.

Szuminksky S, Albers AC, Unger P, Eddy JG. Effect of narrow, pulsed high voltages on bacterial viability. *Phys Ther*. 1994;74(7):660-667.

Chapter Three

Pain Theory and Perception

Learning Objectives

1. Define pain.
2. Discuss chronic and acute pain cycles.
3. Identify the biopsychosocial approach to pain perception.
4. Discuss the pain pathways.
5. List the types and theories of pain and pain management.
6. Describe the importance of assessing pain and its relationship to the clinical reasoning process.

Terminology

Biopsychosocial approach	Pain
Chronic pain	Pain perception
Neurogenic Pain	Referred pain
Nociceptors	Trigger point

Pain

Pain is one of the most frequent ailments for which individuals seek medical attention. Many of the patients seen in occupational therapy report pain as one of the components limiting their ability to actively participate in their occupational roles and tasks. Pain has been characterized as being chronic or acute. *Acute* pain, which lasts from seconds to days, has a biologic function, warning the individual of injury or that something is wrong. *Chronic* pain lacks the biological imperative of acute pain and is pain which recurs at intervals or persists and is of long duration. Chronic pain is often associated with anguish, apprehension, depression, or hopelessness. Pain which is perceived to be in areas other than where the nociceptors (pain receptors) were stimulated is known as referred pain. Low back pain has been described as acute, persistent, and chronic.[1] This model is based on the nature of the symptoms, the patient's response to the symptoms, and the prescribed treatment strategies.

There are a variety of theoretical perspectives of chronic pain, although the majority of the perspectives include the psychological factors of affective, behavioral, cognitive, and sensory-physical.[2-5] Theoretical perspectives on chronic pain have been categorized as *restrictive* and include: mind-body dualism, psychological, radical operant-behavioral, and radical cognitive. Other theoretical perspectives have been categorized as *comprehensive* based on the International Association for the Study of Pain (IASP): gate control, nonradical operant-behavioral, and cognitive-behavioral.[6]

There are many definitions of pain and a variety of clinical phenomena experienced by our patients. Pain has been defined as: the emotion that is the opposite of pleasure,[7] an "emotional experience" caused by tissue injury or described by the patient in terms of tissue damage, or both.[8] The IASP defines pain as an unpleasant sensory or emotional experience which is associated with actual or potential tissue damage or which is described in terms of such damage.[9] Musculoskeletal pain is often the primary complaint of individuals reporting both acute and chronic pain, and is frequently seen in individuals with arthritis.[10,11] Pain occurs when there is a noxious event such as an injury or inflammation to an area of the body. This event or injury causes an excitation of nociceptors in somatic or visceral tissue.

Because pain is such a universal human experience and many of the patients and clients treated by occupational therapists have pain, an understanding of the primary characteristics of pain and interventions which can affect the pain cycle is important. Chronic pain affects all facets of life and society, from its impact on the economy, employment, and health care systems, to the impact on an individual's functional performance in life roles and tasks. By actively treating pain in our patients through the technologies available to us, we are able to more fully integrate our patients into their primary roles and activities, improving outcomes and improving the quality of life.

Biopsychosocial Approach

Pain perception is a multifaceted reaction based on anatomical, physiological, chemical, and psychological factors. These interrelated factors have led to the development of a biopsychosocial approach to the conceptualization and treatment of persistent pain. Biopsychosocial approaches view pain as a complex experience affected by sensory input, but also closely influenced and related to behavioral, cognitive-affective, and environmental factors. These three variables can influence and be influenced by changes in a competing set of variables. The biopsychosocial variables and approach provide a more comprehensive perspective on pain consistent with the underlying values of occupational therapy. For example, a young, newly diagnosed patient with rheumatoid arthritis becomes withdrawn, depressed (a cognitive-behavioral variable), and is in denial (cognitive behavioral variable). She is resistant to help and is unwilling to take her medication which can decrease the disease activity and symptoms (a biological variable). Because of her lack of follow-through and resistance to treatment, she becomes dependent on her spouse, family, and friends (an environmental factor), limiting her occupational behaviors and roles. Because of the influence and dynamic interaction between these competing variables (cognitive-behavioral, biological, and environmental), the patient experiences high levels of pain. [12-13]

To effectively treat the patient with persistent pain, the therapist must recognize the influence and interactions of the factors underlying the biopsychosocial approach and develop strategies and interventions related to each area. The patient and his or her condition must be viewed holistically. Treating the symptom of pain with TENS or other technologies and interventions without addressing the underlying influence of the environmental, cognitive-behavioral, or biological variables and their interaction will result in less than adequate outcomes. TENS can play an important role in the treatment and management of pain, and can be an effective adjunct to conventional occupational therapy intervention. However, to fully enhance the patient's functional independence and outcomes, TENS should never be used in isolation or in place of traditional occupational therapy interventions.

Pain Pathways

Pain is a multidimensional phenomena which profoundly affects an individual psychologically, socioeconomically, and physiologically. Patients experiencing chronic or acute pain may be depressed, anxious, withdrawn, or irritable, and display a variety of maladaptive behavioral responses. Pain is a protective response and is the body's way of informing the individual that something is wrong. The body responds to trauma through a complex series of reactions, including those associated with the sympathetic response of the autonomic nervous system, the "fight-or-flight" response. Nociceptors are receptors located in the skin, viscera, cardiac, and skeletal muscle which receive and transmit painful stimuli.[14-16] Nociceptors may also be affected by the release of endogenous pain-producing substances into the tissue, including potassium, serotonin, bradykinin histamine, prostaglandins, and substance P, which then cause a cascade of effects.[17-18]

Nociceptors are sensory receptors specific to pain that identify potential or actual tissue damage. These receptors are located in the skin, viscera, cardiac and skeletal muscles and respond to different stimulus inputs. Nociceptors are sensitive and responsive to mechanical distortion, variations in the chemical components in the tissue fluid, and by thermal changes. Nociceptors are specialized receptors and possess variable thresholds, some high, some low. Nociceptors respond to the stimulus and signal actual or potential damage to the tissue.[19-20]

Nociceptors carry the action potential by the primary afferent (sensory) neuron, either small myelinated A-delta fibers or small unmyelinated C fibers. The small myelinated A-delta fibers conduct the impulses at a faster rate than the C fibers and stimulation of them may cause a localized sharp "pricking" pain sensation. Stimulation of the unmyelinated C fibers causes a dull, poorly localized burning sensation. Neural activity is carried by these two primary pathways to the higher centers in the brain. The A-delta and C fibers terminate at various levels in the spinal cord in the dorsal horns. Wide-dynamic range neurons and nociceptive-specific neurons receive input from the A-delta and C fibers, assisting in discriminating the type of pain. These wide dynamic range cells are also known as T (transmission) cells.[21-23]

There are several ascending tracts (pathways) which transmit pain signals to the brain. Axons of the majority of the transmission cells cross over, ascending as the lateral spinothalamic tract terminating in the thalamus. This pathway terminates in the portion of the brain known as the somatosensory cortex and perceives pain information as sharp, discriminative, and localized. Other signals are carried by the spinoreticulothalamic pathway which terminates in the reticular formation of the brainstem and thalamus. Axons of this pathway also connect to the midbrain and to structures of the limbic system, basal ganglia and cerebral cortex. This pathway carries information which is perceived as diffuse, poorly localized somatic and visceral pain. [24-29] Descending inhibitory fibers located in the higher brain centers release neurotransmitters, including norepinephrine, serotonin, and enkephalins which moderate and affect the flow of afferent impulses. These inhibitory or descending tracts are activated by endogenous opioids and other neurotransmitters.[30-32]

Types of Pain and Theories

Transcutaneous electrical nerve stimulation (TENS) has been used therapeutically for pain management for approximately 20 years. The IASP has defined pain as an unpleasant sensory and emotional experience associated with actual or potential tissue damage.[33] Though the classification of pain may differ, there are two primary classifications of pain— acute and chronic— though some researchers identify referred pain as a third type. Dependent upon the etiology and clinical manifestations of the condition, each level or type of pain will require a unique therapeutic intervention.

Acute pain has been described as the pain which is most closely associated with tissue damage and nociception. Acute pain usually occurs with a rapid, sudden onset, and is considered a warning signal by the body that tissue damage or injury is about to occur, or has already occurred. There is most often an underlying etiology, and since acute pain signals tissue damage, use of therapeutic physical modalities would be indicated as part of the treatment approach to the condition.[34]

Chronic pain is often poorly localized with the underlying cause not being fully understood or clear to the patient or clinician. Chronic pain is often of long duration, and pervades the individual's life more completely. Physical modalities and technologies are usually ineffective in consistently relieving pain in patients with chronic pain conditions. Persistent pain is pain which continues for long periods of time or is consistently recurrent. Persistent pain is all consuming, affecting all areas of the individual's occupational behaviors. Persistent pain is most effectively treated by limited use of physical agent technologies, with an emphasis placed on behavior modification techniques, patient education, medication, and general conditioning.

Referred pain is pain which is felt at a site different from the original source of the injury or disease. Irritable points in the muscle that referred pain were identified by Travell as "trigger points". A trigger point is a small, localized, hypersensitive area located in the muscle or fascia. Trigger points can be clinically located primarily through palpation. Patients will often be able to localize and identify trigger points when questioned. If the trigger point is stimulated by pressure, heat, or cold, the pain is referred to a remote site. [35-36] Trigger points can be stimulated by acute overload, overwork, fatigue, cooling, and through direct trauma to the muscle. Patients will often report a localized, deep tenderness, often associated with a tight band of skeletal muscle or in the muscle fascia. The trigger point is identifiable as pain upon palpation or compression.

An understanding and identification of the sources of pain are components of effectively utilizing TENS and physical agent technologies. The IASP has identified five different sources of pain: peripheral neurogenic pain, peripheral nociceptive sources of pain, central nervous system-mediated pain, autonomic nervous system mediation of pain, and the affective motivational component. [37]

Peripheral neurogenic pain is caused by the involvement of the neural tissues resulting in mechanical and physiological changes in the body. Clinically, these changes are observed as limitation in movement, pain, paresthesias, or sensory changes. Peripheral nociceptive pain is accompanied by inflammation secondary to the release of chemical mediators such as prostaglandins, histamines, and bradykinins. Peripheral nociceptive pain sources are often the target of involved tissues, and may be mechanical in origin resulting in local dysfunction. The peripheral neurogenic and peripheral nociceptive sources of pain are those most often encountered by the clinician, and respond most successfully to therapeutic intervention and physical agent technologies.

Assessment of Pain

Having a primary understanding of pain-mediation principles facilitates the clinical reasoning process in determining the appropriate intervention for pain control and management. A complete evaluation which assesses pain and function, identifies movement abnormalities, and evaluates anatomical tissue structures assists in identifying realistic treatment goals and interventions.

Pain is a very subjective experience, and clearly identifying the type, location, and sensation of pain in a patient can become problematic. Utilizing both subjective patient descriptions of pain as well as objective measures assists in determining the treatment approach, potential response to intervention, and clinical efficacy. Therapists must also assess the affective motivational component and sources of pain which may influence the evaluation, treatment, prognosis, and outcomes. Aside from the patient's subjective reporting of pain, there are two primary tools which can be used by clinicians to provide a more objective mechanism of reporting—the McGill Pain Questionnaire and Visual Analog Scales.

McGill Pain Questionnaire

The McGill Pain Questionnaire (MPQ) is frequently utilized on initial visits to the clinic. It consists of three parts and includes body diagrams to assist the patient in identifying and locating the area of pain as well as determining whether the pain is internal,

Table 3-1. Pain Scale		
10+	-	Maximal pain
10	-	Very, very strong pain
9	-	
8	-	
7	-	Very strong pain
6	-	
5	-	Strong pain
4	-	Somewhat strong pain
3	-	Moderate pain
2	-	Weak pain
1	-	Very weak pain
0.5	-	Very, very weak pain
0	-	No pain at all

Adapted from Borg, GAV: Psychological basis of perceived exertion. *Med Sci Ex.* 1982; 14: 377-388.

external, or both. The MPQ also includes a Pain Rating Index which consists of a collection of words grouped into categories. The MPQ provides the patient with a method describing the pain and intensity of pain related to activity. Due to the ability to score the MPQ, it provides the clinician with a quantitative method of assessing pain in a patient.[38-42]

Visual Analog Scale

There are several types of pain scales which can provide the clinician with primary information on the patient's response to pain. Utilizing a pain scale provides a mechanism to determine changes and patterns in the level and/or type of pain experienced by the patient. The Visual Analog Scale (VAS) provides the clinician with a quick and relatively accurate method for patients to rate their pain. Visual and analog scales have a 10 cm line marked on a paper with the descriptors: "Pain as bad as it could be" on the left, and "no pain" on the right side of the line. Patients are asked to mark along the line to indicate the amount or intensity of pain they are experiencing. This scale can be administered before and after treatment sessions, and the therapist measures the distance along the continuum to provide a method of rating the patient's response. Because of the ease of application, if used consistently, the VAS can assist the clinician in monitoring patient progress and response to treatment interventions (Table 3-1).

Summary

An understanding and appreciation of pain in our patients provides the clinician with an additional clue in the clinical reasoning process. Pain is a component of many of the soft tissue injuries which can be treated with physical agent technologies. Along with pain, the patient may display any number of occupational performance components, including altered sensation, edema, muscle guarding, weakness, or loss of movement. Recognizing pain patterns associated with different sources of pain, and understanding the patient's altered biomechanics and musculoskeletal compensations will facilitate treatment outcomes and enhance appropriate occupational interventions.[43]

References

1. DeRosa CP, Porterfield JA. A physical therapy model for the treatment of low back pain. *Phys Ther*. 1992;72:261-272.

2. Fordyce WE. *Behavior Methods for Chronic Pain and Illness*. St Louis, MO: C.V. Mosby; 1976.

3. Melzack R, Torgerson WS. On the language of pain. *Anesthesiology*. 1971;34:50.

4. Melzack R, Wall P. *The Challenge of Pain*. New York: Penguin Books; 1982.

5. Altmairer EM, Lehmann TR, Russel DW, Weinstein JN, Kao CF. The effectiveness of psychological interventions for the rehabilitation of low back pain: a randomized controlled trial evaluation. *Pain*. 1992;49;329-335.

6. Novy DM, Nelson DV, Francis DJ. Perspectives of chronic pain: An evaluative comparison of restrictive and comprehensive models. *Psychological Bulletin*. 1995;118:2,238-247.

7. Sweet WH. *Pain-Handbook of Physiology*. 1927;1:14-19,1959.

8. Steinbach RA. *Pain-A Psychophysiological Analysis*. New York: Academic Press; 1968: 11-12.

9. Hakim MH. Pain and its measurement. *Hamdard*. 1995;38:86-90.

10. Kazis LE, Meenan RF, Anderson JJ. Pain in the rheumatic diseases: investigations of a key health status component. *Arthritis Rheum*. 1983;26(8):1017-1022.

11. Keefe FJ, Egert J. A cognitive-behavioral perspective on patients with cumulative trauma disorders. In: Sauter SL, Moon SD, eds. *Psychosocial Aspects of Musculoskeletal Disorders in Office Work*. Durham, NC: Taylor & Francis (in press).

12. Fordyce WE. *The biopsychosocial model revisited*. Presented at the annual meeting of the American Pain Society, Los Angeles, CA: November, 1995.

13. Keefe F, Kashikar-Zuck S, et al. Pain in arthritis and musculoskeletal disorders: the role of coping skills training and exercise interventions. *JOSPT*. 1996;24:279-290.

14. Bonica JJ. *The Management of Pain, Vols I and II*. 2nd ed. Malvern, PA: Lea & Febiger; 1990.

15. Sherrington CS. *The Integrative Action of the Nervous System*. New York: Scribner; 1906.

16. Anderson KV, Parl GS. *Long term increases in nociceptive threshold following lesions in feline nucleus reticularis gigantocellularis (abst)*. 1st World Congress on Pain. 1975;1:70.

17. Hanegan JL. Principles of nociception. In: Gersh MR. *Electrotherapy in Rehabilitation*. Philadelphia, Pa: FA Davis; 1992:26.

18. Perl ER. Characteristics of nociceptors and their activation of neurons in the superficial dorsal horn: first steps for the sensation of pain. In: Kruger L and Liebeskind JC (eds). *Advances in Pain Research and Therapy*, Vol 6. New York: Raven Press; 1984:23.

19. Torebjork HE, Hallin RG. Perceptual changes accompanying controlled preferential blocking of A and C fibre responses in intact human skin nerves. *Exp Brain Res*. 1973;16:321.

20. Kerr FWL. An overview of neural mechanisms of pain. *Neurosci Res Program Bull*. 1978;16:30.

21. Dubner R, Bennett GJ. Spinal and trigeminal mechanisms of nociception. *Annu Rev Neurosci*. 1983;6:381.

22. LaMotte RH. Peripheral neural mechanisms of cutaneous hyperalgesia following mild injury by heat. *J Neurosci.* 1982;2:765.

23. Kandel ER, Schwartz JH, Jessel TM. *Principles of Neural Science. 3rd ed.* New York: Elsevier; 1991.

24. Willis WD. *The Pain System.* New York: S Karger; 1985:264.

25. Hanegan JL. Principles of nociception. In: Gersh MR, ed. *Electrotherapy in Rehabilitation.* Philadelphia, PA: F.A. Davis; 1992:26.

26. Rodbard S. Pain associated with muscular activity. *Am Heart J.* 1975:90:84-92.

27. Melzack R, Wall PD. Pain mechanisms: a new theory. *Science.* 1965;150:971.

28. Wall PD. Modulation of pain by painful and nonpainful events. In: Bonica JJ and Able-Fessard D, eds. *Advances in Pain Research and Therapy, Vol 1.* New York: Raven Press;1976:1.

29. Charman RA. Pain theory and physiotherapy. *Physiotherapy.* 1989;75;5:247-254.

30. Bennet GJ. Neuropathic pain. In: Wall PD, Melzack R, eds. *Textbook of Pain.* 3rd ed. Edinburgh: Churchill Livingstone;1994:201-224.

31. D'Amours R, Ferrante F. Postoperative pain management. *JOSPT.* 1996;24:227-236.

32. International Association for the Study of Pain, IASP *Subcommittee on Taxonomy*, 1986.

33. Fedorczyk J. The role of physical agents in modulating pain. *J Hand Ther.* 1997;10:110-121.

34. Travell J. Myofascial trigger points: Clinical view. In Bonica JJ and Able-Fessard DG, eds. *Advances in Pain Research and Therapy, Vol.2.* New York: Raven Press; 1976:919.

35. Travell JG, Simons DG. *Myofascial Trigger Point Manual.* Baltimore, MD: Williams & Wilkins; 1982.

36. Ohnhaus EE, Adler R. Methodological problems in the measurement of pain: a comparison between the verbal rating scale and the visual analogue scale. *Pain.* 1975;1:379.

37. Price DD, Harkins SW. Combined use of experimental pain and visual analogue scales in providing standardized measurements of clinical pain. *Clin J Pain.* 1987;3:1.

38. Melzack R. The McGill Pain Questionnaire: major properties and scoring methods. *Pain.* 1975;1:277.

39. Kelpac RK. Sensitivity of the McGill Pain Questionnaire to intensity and quality of laboratory pain. *Pain.* 1981;10:199.

40. Bryne M. Cross validation of the factor structure of MPQ. *Pain.* 1982;13:193.

41. Bowsher D. Acute and chronic pain and assessment. In: Wells PE, Frampton V, Bowsher D, eds. *Pain Management in Physical Therapy.* Norwalk, CT: Appleton & Lange; 1988:39-44.

42. Fleetwood-Walker SM, Mitchell R, Hope PJ, et al. An a2 receptor mediates the selective inhibition by nonadrenaline of nociceptive responses of identified dorsal horn neurons. *Brain Res.* 1985;334:243-254.

Bibliography

Caudill M, Holman G, Turk D. Effective ways to manage chronic pain. *Patient Care.* 1996;154-172.

Mannheimer JS, Lampe GN. *Clinical Transcutaneous Electrical Nerve Stimulation.* Philadelphia, Pa: F.A. Davis; 1984.

Melzack R, Wall P. Pain mechanisms: a new theory. *Science.* 1965;150:971-977.

Mersky H, Bogduk N. *Classification of Chronic Pain.* 2nd ed. Seattle, Wash: IASP Press; 1994.

Ruda MA, Bennett GJ, Dubner R. Neurochemistry and neurocircuitry in the dorsal horn. *Prog Brain Res.* 1986;66:219-268.

Salar G, Job I, Mingrino S, et al. Effect of transcutaneous electrotherapy on CSF betaendorphin content in patients without pain problems. *Pain.* 1984;10:169-172.

Tyrer SR, ed. *Psychology, Psychiatry and Chronic Pain.* Oxford: Butterworth and Heinemann; 1992.

Walsh M, Muntzer E. Hand therapists are you prepared? *Rehab 2.* 1996; 49-53.

Chapter Four

Cryotherapy

Learning Objectives

1. Describe the application techniques for cold modalities.
2. Discuss the types of cold agents available.
3. Identify the biophysiological changes which occur with cryotherapy.
4. Discuss the clinical reasoning involved in application of cold agents.
5. Identify the precautions and indications for the application of cold.

Terminology

Conduction	Hyperemia
Cryoglobulinemia	Ice Massage
Cryotherapy	Superficial Cooling
Evaporation	Vapocoolant

Cryotherapy or cold therapy is a common modality frequently used by therapists in the treatment of acute injuries or trauma, for decreasing spasticity and spasms, and in reducing edema. Cryotherapy is the application of any substance to the body which results in a withdrawal of heat from the body, effectively lowering the temperature of the tissue. Cryotherapy has been used in medicine since the ancient Greeks, and derives its name from the Greek word for cold, *cryos*. When used therapeutically, superficial cold techniques exert their effect on the tissue to depths of 1 to 2 cm. As with any other physical technology, cryotherapy is most effectively used as an adjunct to the treatment process.

There are a number of techniques and methods of applying cold agents to tissue, including ice massage, cold or ice packs, cold baths, cold compression units, and vapo-coolant sprays. Transmission of cooling occurs through the mechanisms of conduction and evaporation. When the source of the cold is in direct contact with the tissue surface, and there is a difference in the temperature between the source and the tissue surface, energy is transferred through conduction.[1] Evaporation occurs when a liquid is changed to a gas. This change from liquid to gas requires energy in the form of heat to occur. In the use of vapocoolant sprays, the heat necessary to produce this change comes from the skin surface, which effectively cools the tissue.

Superficial cooling of the tissue lowers tissue temperature to varying degrees and is most often used with neuromuscular and musculoskeletal conditions, and following an acute injury. Superficial cold lowers the tissue temperature and can produce analgesia, decrease edema, reduce muscle spasm, and lower metabolic activity. Temperature change and biophysical effects of cooling are related to the time of exposure, the method used to cool the tissue, and the conductivity of the tissue. Deeper subcutaneous tissue such as muscles and joints will require a longer exposure to the agent in order to affect biophysical changes in the tissue. The type of tissue and depth of the tissue also influence the biophysical changes and length of time needed to cool the tissue, dependent on the thermal conductivity of the tissue. Thermal conductivity refers to the efficiency of a tissue to conduct heat. Muscle, which has a high water content, conducts heat more efficiently than adipose or fat tissue, which acts as an insulator.[2,3] Obese patients may not achieve the same biophysical effects when cold is applied, requiring longer exposure time to the intervention. Caution needs to be used, however, when considering the length of exposure to the cold agent. Changes in the skin's temperature occur very quickly, and damage to the skin and tissue may occur before the desired biophysical effects are achieved.

Cryotherapy Effects

Superficial cooling of the temperature may produce analgesia, a reduction in edema, decrease in muscle spasm, and a reduction in the metabolic activity of the tissue. Application of cold has a direct effect on the nerves and nerve endings, causing an analgesic effect through counter irritation, and by reducing the metabolic activity of the tissue.[4] All nerve fibers are impacted by the application of cold, but small, myelinated pain fibers are the first to be affected by the cold. As temperature is decreased, there is a concurrent reduction in nerve conduction velocities along with a decrease in acetylcholine production. As the exposure to cold is lengthened, there is a concomitant increase in the recovery cycle of the nerve following excitation, along with an increase in the refractory period.[5]

The analgesic effect of cryotherapy can be used to the therapist's advantage by involving the patient in activities and occupations which may have been limited due to the pain. The analgesic effect of cold intervention may also decrease a patient's need for pain medication, and care must be taken to monitor the activity level to ensure that further trauma does not occur through overuse.[6]

Cold can also cause a decrease in edema in some patients. Application of cold causes vasoconstriction by sympathetic reflex and through its effect on the smooth muscle of the blood vessels. Reduction of edema appears to be most effective when combined with compression.[7,8] Vasoconstriction of the arterioles and venules occurs following application of cold for 15 minutes or less. In patients with acute trauma, application of cold is most effective when combined with compression and elevation.[9,10] To lower the possibility of thermal damage to postoperative patients, application of a less intense cold three to four times daily for 20 to 30 minutes, in combination with compression and elevation, should be considered.

Cold's effect on the muscle spindle mechanism and sensory wrappings of the spindle mechanism causes a decrease in muscle spasm. Muscle spasm and the associated pain often limit range of motion, and function negatively, impacting occupational performance. Use of cold packs or ice massage may be an effective intervention to decrease the spasm and to improve range of motion when combined with static positional stretch or contract-relax techniques. Cooling the tissue causes a slowing of muscle contraction and relaxation.[11-13] If muscles are cooled to a temperature less than 80°F, grip strength and sustained contraction become reduced. Engaging a patient in activities that require fine motor control may be contraindicated following application of cold due to the decreased performance secondary to the biophysical changes of the tissue.[14-16] Application of 10 minutes of cryotherapy may be enough to decrease muscle spasm in most individuals, though an obese client with greater amounts of adipose tissue may require up to 30 minutes to achieve the same effect.

Intraarticular enzymatic activity is decreased following application of cold. Reduction of metabolic activity can reduce energy requirements which may facilitate and account, in part, for cold's effectiveness in the acute phase of injuries. Because of its biophysical effects on the healing process, cold is the thermal intervention which should be used following an acute injury (24 to 48 hours). Applying cold to the area immediately following injury will decrease pain, inflammation, edema, and muscle spasm. Use of cryotherapy as part of the treatment protocol in treating musculoskeletal trauma and postorthopedic surgical swelling and pain is well documented. Benefits of applying cold after injury or surgery include a reduction in the need for pain medication, decreased pain, decreased edema, improved ROM, decreased spasm, reduction of exercise induced muscle soreness, and quicker return to activity.[17-22]

Indications

The most common use for cryotherapy is in the treatment of acute injury and inflammation, 24-48 hours post injury. Other conditions and indications for the use of cold include:
- · edema (combined with compression, exercise, or massage)
- · post exercise edema and pain
- · arthritic flare-up

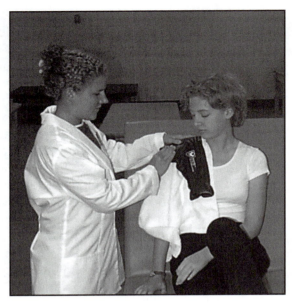

Figure 4-1. Cold application using a commercial cold pack. The cold pack can also be placed in a pillowcase. Skin condition should be monitored.

• acute bursitis or tendinitis
• spasticity
• acute or chronic pain secondary to muscle spasm
• after exercise to maintain soft tissue elongation

The standard protocol of rest, ice, compression, and elevation (RICE) is effective in decreasing the effects of acute musculoskeletal trauma. Cold should be applied to the injured area for 20 minutes per half hour to 30 minutes per 2 hours for the first 6 to 24 hours after trauma. Spasticity requires a cooling period of between 10 to 20 minutes before spastic muscle decreases in tone facilitating movement.

Cold Application

There are a number of methods and techniques which can be used in the treatment application of cold. These include cold packs, ice massage, cold/ice water immersion baths, cool whirlpools, ice towels, and vapocoolant sprays. Patients will feel a variety of sensations when applying cold. The intensity and rapidity of the sensation may be dependent upon the mechanism of application used. The initial stage of cooling is marked by intense cold with skin reddening (hyperemia), followed by a burning sensation, then a deep aching feeling, leading ultimately to analgesia, which occurs 10-20 minutes after beginning cryotherapy (Figure 4-1).

Cold Packs

Cold packs are available commercially or can very easily be made at home using either a homemade alcohol pack, crushed ice in a plastic bag, or simply using a frozen bag of peas. Cold packs are an effective and inexpensive method for administering cold to an area. An advantage to using cold packs is the ability of the pack to conform to the extremity or area which is being treated. Use of cold packs is also advantageous because the therapist can target large or multiple areas for treatment, and combine elevation and icing to facilitate edema reduction.

When used for musculoskeletal injuries, the cold pack should ideally cover the entire muscle from origin to insertion, though this is not always possible. The cold pack can be applied directly to the area, or it may be wrapped in a wet or dry towel or a pillowcase and then applied. An insulating material should always be used when the ice pack is placed over a bony prominence. If a distal extremity such as a hand, wrist, or elbow is the targeted tissue, the extremity can be covered with an Ace wrap (Bergen Brunswig, Orange, CA), compression wrap such as Tubigrip (Tubition House, Oldham, England), or Stockinette (Smith and Nephew, Germantown, WI), followed by the placement of wet or dry cloth towels or paper towels acting as an interface between the tissue and the cold pack. Ace wraps or other elastic type wraps such as Coban (3M Healthcare, St. Paul, MN) tape can be used to maintain and hold the position of the cold pack on the area being treated. Cold packs can be left on for an average treatment time of 10-20 minutes with close monitoring of the skin to prevent tissue damage from too rapid or prolonged cooling.

Ice Massage

Ice massage is the application of ice on the skin or targeted area of treatment and is most often used to anesthetize an area or to apply cold to a trigger point. Because the ice is applied directly to the skin, smaller, localized areas are more effectively treated. As with any cryotherapy application, the size of the area to be treated and the amount of adipose, or fat tissue, needs to be taken into consideration before applying the intervention. Ice cubes or water placed in a paper or foam cup and frozen are the most frequently used methods, though commercial cryo-probes are available. The patient should be positioned comfortably with the area to be treated exposed and draped with a towel to absorb the melting water. The ice cube or cup is slowly rubbed in small, rhythmical circles, maintaining direct contact with the skin at all times. The patient should be informed of the stages of cold, burning, and aching, followed by numbness, and repeatedly questioned to identify which stage of cooling is occurring. When the patient reports numbness or lost feeling of touch, it is generally safe to continue for approximately 1 more minute. Ice massage should rarely exceed 7 minutes in length; most often treatment should last from approximately 3-10 minutes depending on the size of the area being treated.[23,24]

Cold/Ice Water Immersion Baths & Cool Whirlpool

Use of cold water baths or cool whirlpools are most often used for edema reduction and used in conjunction with string wrapping or compression wrapping, eg, for digital or hand injuries. An advantage to the use of cold or ice baths is the fact that there is complete contact of the cooling agent on the tissue being treated because the extremity is immersed completely in water. Cool whirlpools can be effective in facilitating wound debridement, secondary to the agitation of the water, particularly in a hand injury which may be edematous. When used in upper extremity injuries, a disadvantage to the use of cold or ice baths and whirlpools is the dependent position of the hand and extremity. Patients should be advised to continue hand pumping and exercise throughout the treatment, including periodic elevation of the extremity above the level of their heart with the pumping of the hand, to facilitate venous return. Therapeutic water temperatures may be between 35-75° F, or 13-18° C. Treatment duration is between 15-20 minutes, though colder temperatures will require a corresponding decrease in duration.

Ice Towels

Ice towels are another mechanism for draping the cold around the targeted area. Ice towels may contain ice chips or shavings, or may be dipped in ice water, wrung out and wrapped around an extremity. Because the towels cool quickly, they will need to be changed frequently, often every 5-6 minutes. An advantage to the use of ice towels is the ability to circumferentially cover an extremity, and as such they may be more effective than other mechanisms at reducing spasticity. Conversely, they melt quickly, and may prove to be uncomfortable for the patient and the therapist due to the melting water, discomfort to the patient, and inconvenience.

Cold Compression Units

Cold compression units, such as the Cryotemp from Jobst Corporation, are refrigerated units that circulate cooled water over an extremity and are similar in principle to the workings of a refrigerator or freezer cooling unit. The temperature can be adjusted by the therapist and can remain constant throughout the length of the treatment. The cooled medium is circulated through a sleeve or garment which surrounds the targeted extremity. Cold compression units combine an edema compression pump with the advantages of cold and may be effective at edema reduction. They are often used for treating a variety of musculoskeletal injuries. Most patients are able to tolerate 50° F for 15-20 minutes. A disadvantage to the use of cold compression units is the cost of the equipment, and care must be taken with regard to the amount of pressure applied, and which may be contraindicated in the treatment diagnosis.

Vapocoolant Sprays

Vapocoolant sprays were initially used in the treatment of trigger points, with Travell developing the "stretch and spray" technique.[25] There have been two commercially available sprays, ethyl chloride and Fluori-Methane. Ethyl chloride is a local anesthetic but is flammable and volatile, and may explode if heated or dropped. Flouri-Methane spray contained a fluorocarbon which was banned in January of 1996 due to the Clean Air Act of 1990 limiting the release of fluorocarbons in the environment.[26] Vapocoolant sprays contain a liquid which is under pressure. This chemical is sprayed on the tissue coming into contact with the area of the skin being treated. Due to its chemical composition and properties, the chemical evaporates, cooling the skin for short periods of time. The spray can be applied to a trigger point area, or to the entire length of the muscle in a sweeping, unidirectional motion with the muscle being positioned in a passive stretch.[27] Vapocoolant sprays are used by many athletes and may be effective in the treatment of acute muscle spasms. However, their effectiveness may be relatively short lived (10-15 minutes), and the spray is expensive.[28] In addition, the technique is very therapist dependent, requiring direct contact and support of the therapist throughout the intervention.

Precautions

Cold is an effective intervention with physiological effects which can last several hours. Rewarming of the tissue takes approximately 20 minutes, and though cold is rel-

Table 4-1.
Cryotherapy Precautions

· Monitor blood pressure, since cold can cause a temporary increase in systolic and diastolic blood pressure

· Avoid use in patients with impaired circulation or hypersensitivity to cold

· Avoid application directly over wounds which are 2-3 weeks post injury

· Avoid prolonged placement over superficial nerve

Always monitor patient's skin condition

atively easy to apply and is indicated in a number of treatment conditions, care should always be used in its application, and skin condition should be monitored closely.

A cold gel pack should never be directly placed on the skin because the temperatures at the skin interface can be subfreezing. Application of the cold pack should never last longer than 20 minutes. Aside from their volatility, caution should be used with vapocoolant sprays because they can freeze the skin on contact. When the patient reports numbness, indicating analgesia, the patient's protective sensation is removed and the patient should be cautioned against overuse or reinjury to the area. In distal extremities such as hands, edema may result if cryotherapy is too severe. This may be due in part to the increased permeability of the lymph vessels.

Cold should not be used in patients with specific cold-sensitivity, such as cold urticaria, cryoglobulinemia, and Raynaud's disease. Sensitivity to the cold may be indicated by the development of itching, hives, or sweating, with the development of wheals with reddened borders and blanched centers.[29,30] Patients with cold urticaria may also develop a massive histamine release and subsequent systemic reactions including increased heart rate, decreased blood pressure, and syncope. Cryoglobulinemia is characterized by an abnormal blood protein which forms a gel when it is exposed to cold.[31] Patients with Raynaud's phenomenon may have episodes of pallor, cyanosis, rubor, numbness, tingling, or burning to the digits. Cold should never be applied to areas of compromised circulation, such as peripheral vascular disease, patients with hypertension, or to patients who have had frostbite in the area which is being treated.

Though cold is easily and safely applied, patients should always be monitored closely for reactions to the treatment. Any form of cryotherapy should never be used for longer than 1 continuous hour, and skin condition and patient's response should always be monitored. Documentation should always include the treatment parameters, including duration, site of application, and method used to apply the cold. Other considerations include the patient's response to the treatment and any changes or revisions to the patient goals. Any changes in the patient's occupational performance abilities should also be documented (Table 4-1).

Case Study

This is a 38-year-old right hand dominant female with primary complaint of pain in the left elbow with recent onset of 24 hours. She states that she "banged the outside" of her elbow against the doorframe when carrying groceries into her house. She reports "constant" pain in the elbow; and rates the pain as a 6-7/10, with magnification of the pain with use. She describes the pain as radiating down toward her fingers and is unable to lift heavy objects.

Examination of the elbow and the proximal posterior forearm reveal temperature variation, with the area warmer to the touch than the noninvolved side. Circumferential measurements are greater on the affected side. ROM measurements are WNLs, though movements are guarded. There is point tenderness over the lateral epicondylitis and pain associated with the wrist loaded in extension. Grip and pinch strengths are decreased secondary to pain. There is discoloration with bruising noted at the elbow where the impact occurred. Treatment goals are to decrease pain, improve pain-free ROM, and improve strength. Initial treatment protocol includes application of an ice pack to the affected area. The patient is also instructed in a home exercise program (HEP) of icing to the area. Three MHz ultrasound at 20% duty cycle at .2W/cm2 for 5 minutes is also used as part of the treatment to decrease the inflammatory process. Monitoring the patient's HEP and compliance is crucial to determine any changes to the goals and treatment protocol. Engagement in occupational activities requiring gentle flexion and extension to the elbow are also included in the protocol after the physical agents.

References

1. McMaster WC. Cryotherapy. *Physician Sports Med*. 1982;10(11):113-119.

2. Hecox B, Fond D. *Physical Agents*. Norwalk, Conn: Appleton & Lange; 1994.

3. Wolf SL, Basmajian JV. Intramuscular temperature changes deep to localized cutaneous cold stimulation. *Phys Ther*. 1973;53:1284.

4. Lehmann JF, Masock AJ, Warren CG, et al. Effect of therapeutic temperatures on tendon extensibility. *Arch Phys Med Rehabil*. 1970;51(8):481-487.

5. Lehmann JF, ed. *Therapeutic Heat and Cold* 4th ed. Baltimore, Md: Williams & Wilkins; 1990.

6. Cohn BT, Draeger RI, Jackson DW. The effects of cold therapy in the postoperative management of pain in patients undergoing anterior cruciate ligament reconstruction. *Am J Sports Med*. 1989;17(3):344-349.

7. Sloan JP, Giddings P, Hain R. Effects of cold and compression on edema. *Phys Sportsmed*. 1988;16(8):116-120.

8. Conolly WB, Paltos N, Tooth RM. Cold therapy-An improved method. *Med J Aust*. 1972;2:42.

9. Levy AS, Marmar E. The role of cold compression dressings in the postoperative treatment of total knee arthroplasty. *Clin Orthop*. 1993;297:174.

10. Healy WI, Seidman J, Pfeiffer BA, Brown DG. Cold compressive dressing after total knee arthroplasty. *Clin Orthop*. 1994;299:143.

11. Major TC, Schwainghamer JM, Winston S. Cutaneous and skeletal muscle vascular responses to hypothermia. *Am J Physiol*. 1981;240(6).

12. Zankel HT. Effect of physical agents on motor conduction velocity of the ulnar nerve. *Arch Phys Med Rehabil*. 1966;47:787.

13. Hedenberg L. Functional improvement of the spastic hemiplegic arm after cooling. *Scand J Rehabil Med*. 1970;2:154.

14. Johnson J, Leider FE. Influence of cold bath on maximum handgrip strength. *Percept Mot Skills*. 1977;44:323.

15. Thompson G. Effect of cryotherapy on eccentric peak torque and endurance (abstract). *Journal of Athletic Training*. 1944;29:180.

16. Knight KL. The effects of cold application on nerve conduction velocity and muscle force (abstract). *Journal of Athletic Training*. 1997;332:5.

17. Hocutt JE, Jaffe R, Rylander CR, Beebe JK. Cryotherapy in ankle sprains. *Am J Sports Med*. 1982;10:316.

18. Benson TB, Copp EP. The effects of therapeutic forms of heat and ice on the pain threshold of normal shoulder. *Rheumatol Rehabil*. 1974;13:101.

19. Grant AE. Massage with ice (cryokinetics) in the treatment of painful conditions of the musculoskeletal system. *Arch Phys Med Rehabil*. 1964;45:233.

20. Prentice, WE. An electromyographic analysis of the effectiveness of heat or cold and stretching for inducing relaxation in injured muscle. *J Orthop Sports Phys Ther*. 1982;3:133.

21. Yackszn L, Adams C, Francis KT. The effects of ice massage on delayed muscle soreness. *Am J Sports Med*. 1984;12:159.

22. Knight KL. *Cryotherapy: Theory, Technique, Physiology*. Chattanooga, TN: Chattanooga Corp; 1985.

23. Lowdon BJ, Moore RJ. Determinants and nature of intramuscular temperature change during cold therapy. *J Phys Med*. 1975;54:223-233.

24. Waylonis GW. The physiologic effect of ice massage. *Arch Phys Med Rehabil*. 1967;48:37.

25. Travell JG, Simons DG. *Myofascial Pain and Dysfunction: The Trigger Point Manual*. 2nd ed. Baltimore, MD: Williams and Wilkins; 1992.

26. Clean Air Act of 1991, *Federal Register*, January 1, 1996.

27. Travell JG, Simons DG. *Myofascial Pain and Dysfunction: The Trigger Point Manual*. Baltimore, MD: Williams & Wilkins; 1983.

28. Simons D, Travell J. Myofascial trigger points: a possible explanation. *Pain*. 1981;10:106-109.

29. Shelley WB, Crao WA. Cold erythema: A new hypersensitivity syndrome. *JAMA*. 1962;180:639.

30. Day MJ. Hypersensitive response to ice massage: Report of a case. *Phys Ther*. 1974;54:592.

31. Schumacher HR ed. Cryoglobulinemia. In: Shumacher HR, Klippel JH, Robinson DR. *Primer on Rheumatic Diseases*. 9th ed. Atlanta, Ga: Arthritis Foundation; 1988:82.

Bibliography

Abramson DI. Changes in blood flow, oxygen uptake and tissue temperatures produced by the topical application of wet heat. *Arch Phys Med Rehabil*. 1961;42:305.

Behnke R. Cold therapy. *Athlet Train*. 1974;9:178.

Belitsky RB, Odam SJ, Hubley-Kozey C. Evaluation of the effectiveness of wet ice, dry ice, and Cryogen packs in reducing skin temperature. *Phys Ther*. 1987;67:1090.

Bugaj R. The cooling, analgesic, and rewarming effects of ice massage on localized skin. *Phys Ther*. 1975;55:11.

Downey JA. Physiologic effects of heat and cold. *J Am Phys Ther Assoc*. 1964;44:713.

Green GA, Zachazewski JE, Jordan SE. A case conference: peroneal nerve palsy induced bycryotherapy. *Physician and Sports Medicine*. 1989;17:63.

Greenspan JD, Taylor DJ, McGillis SL. Body site variation of cool perception thresholds, with observations on paradoxical heat. *Somatosens Mot Res*. 1993;10:467.

Ho SS. Comparison of various icing times in decreasing bone metabolism and blood flow in the knee. *Am J Sports Med*. 1995;23:74.

Ingersoll CD, Mangus BC. Sensations of cold reexamined: a study using the McGill Pain Questionnaire. *Athletic Training*. 1991;26:240.

Knight KL. Circulatory effects of therapeutic cold applications. In: Knight KL, ed. *Cryotherapy in Sport Injury Management*. Champaign, IL: Human Kinetics; 1995:107-125.

Levy AS, Marmar E. The role of cold compression dressings in the postoperative treatment of total knee arthroplasty. *Clin Orthop and Rel Res*. 1993;297:174.

Miglietta O. Action of cold on spasticity. *Am J Phys Med*. 1973;52:198.

Murphy AJ. The physiological effects of cold application. *Phys Ther Rev*. 1960;40:1112.

Olsen JE, Stravino U. A review of cryotherapy. *Phys Ther*. 1972;52:840.

Waylonis GW. The physiologic effect of ice massage. *Arch Phys Med Rehabil*.1967;48:37.

Wessman MS, Kottke FJ. The effect of indirect heating on peripheral blood flow, pulse rate, blood pressure and temperature. *Arch Phys Med Rehabil*. 1967;48:567.

Chapter Five

Superficial Heat Agents

Don Earley, MA, OTR

Learning Objectives

1. Define SHAs.
2. Differentiate between conduction and convection.
3. Discuss the synergy of heat and therapeutic occupation.
4. Discuss the factors that influence tissue temperature elevation.
5. Differentiate between mild, moderate, and vigorous dosages of heat.
6. Discuss the biophysical effects of heat.
7. Specify the indications for and precautions or contraindications of using SHAs.
8. Demonstrate clinical reasoning in the selection of SHAs.
9. Discuss the clinical applications of hydrotherapy, fluidotherapy, hot pack, contrast bath, warm water soak, and paraffin.

Terminology

Active Modality	Mild Dose
Conduction	Moderate Dose
Convection	Superficial Heat Agents
Dependent Limb Position	Systemic Effects
Local Effects	Vigorous Effects
Passive Modality	

Superficial heat agents (SHAs) are defined as the therapeutic application of any modality to the skin which results in an increased skin and superficial subcutaneous tissue temperature.[1] Superficial heat is primarily transmitted through conduction and convection. Conduction is the exchange of thermal energy between two surfaces in physical contact, such as with a hot pack, contrast bath, or paraffin. Convection is the conveyance of heat by the movement of heated particles. Air or water molecules move across the body part being treated, creating temperature variations.[2] Physical agents such as whirlpool bath or fluidotherapy use convection to heat tissue.

Superficial heat agents increase the superficial tissue temperature to varying degrees depending on the intensity of the heat, the medium used, time of exposure, and the surface area involved. Superficial heat typically has a therapeutic effect at depths of up to 1 cm.[3] At 1 cm, tissue temperature is raised by an average of 6° F, and at 2 cm, it is raised approximately 2° F.[4,5]

Basic Principles

Research studies support the union of superficial heat and occupation. Greenburg[6], in a study investigating superficial heat and activity on local blood flow, found that activity was the best way to increase blood flow. Greenburg's results also indicated that heat and activity together produced blood flow three times greater than just heat or activity alone. For many of our patients, however, activity performance is limited due to their injuries. SHAs may be used to facilitate their performance. Incorporating SHAs into the treatment process sets the stage for functional activity and associated movement. Lehman[7] noted that superficial heat application prior to passive or active mobilization procedures required less force to obtain connective tissue elongation and improve tissue viscoelasticity. Lehman further demonstrated that temperature elevation without stress produced no therapeutic extensibility of tissue. Norkin and Levangie[8] state that changes in tissue temperature affect the rate of creep or deformation of tissue. The mechanism of creep, or tissue elongation, is via heat and therapeutic occupation. These studies demonstrate that modalities in conjunction with occupation may produce maximal effects and benefits for some patients. The research supports a fundamental principle that for some diagnoses and conditions, heat is physiologically advantageous to the target tissues, and ultimately to the patient's occupational performance.

Physiological Response to Temperature Variation

An understanding of the physiological responses to temperature variation before using a heat or thermal agent for therapeutic intervention is necessary to appropriately and effectively select the correct method and agent. The temperature dosage must be considered when selecting a SHA. Safe dosages involve a subcutaneous tissue temperature rise of 0-14° F.[9,10] The physiologic response is dependent on the extent of the temperature elevation within the tissue. Elevation of tissue temperature is also dependent on the rate that the selected temperature is added to the tissue, the duration of tissue temperature elevation, and the volume of tissue exposed.[11] Conduction is also a factor influencing the physiological response. If moist heat is used, conduction will be influenced by application procedures, such as draping the hot pack over a body part or resting the weighted body part over the hot pack. These factors need to be considered when selecting an appropriate heat agent because there is no objective manner by which to determine the exact dosage. If tissue temperatures elevate to levels greater than desired, one must reconsider such factors as the selected modality temperature and the rate at which the heat is being delivered. There are three primary levels of heat delivery to achieve tissue temperature elevation: mild, moderate, and vigorous dosage.

A mild dose implies that only a slight change in tissue temperature is noted, with the primary benefits related to the sensation of warmth. A dry heating pad or warm water soaks used for short periods at home are two examples of delivering a mild dose to the tissue. Hydrotherapy used to facilitate wound healing is another example. A moderate dose implies an increase in tissue temperature to approximately 102-106° F, with only a slight increase in blood flow. This dosage is typically used when heat is indicated, yet the potential for edema is a concern. A vigorous dose implies a marked increase in blood flow with a tissue temperature rise of 107-113° F.[12] This dosage may be beneficial to ischemic conditions and is typically used when heat is indicated, yet edema is not a concern.

The SHAs provided within the clinical setting are typically capable of providing moderate and vigorous dosages. A subcutaneous tissue temperature elevation to 113°F or higher can be unsafe and may cause damage. [13] When heat is applied, the vascular protective response of vasodilation occurs. This assists in the regulation and removal of heat from the body. If the temperature of the tissues rises faster than the body can dissipate the heat, tissue temperature increases. This becomes unsafe at temperatures exceeding 113° F, and damage to the tissue may occur.

Biophysical Effects

There are four primary effects of SHAs: analgesic, vascular, metabolic, and connective tissue responses.

Analgesic effects of heat involve reducing pain symptomatology. Heat acts selectively on free nerve endings, tissues, and peripheral nerve fibers, either directly or indirectly, reducing pain and elevating pain tolerance.[14,15] When the level of pain a person is experiencing decreases, there may be a concurrent improvement in functional outcomes and performance. To achieve analgesic effects, a mild, moderate or vigorous dose of heat may be considered.

The vascular effects of heat can aid in pain relief and in decreasing muscle spasm. A 6-14° F tissue temperature rise facilitates the release of substances, such as histamines, into the bloodstream, resulting in vasodilation. This increase in blood flow reduces ischemia, muscle spindle activity and tonic muscle contractions, thereby reducing pain.[1] To achieve vascular effects, a moderate to vigorous dose of heat should be considered.

The metabolic effects of heat can aid in pain relief and tissue repair. Increased blood flow and oxygen within the tissue bring greater numbers of antibodies, leukocytes, nutrients, and enzymes to injured tissues. Pain is reduced by the removal of byproducts of the inflammatory process. Nutrition is enhanced at the cellular level and cellular repair occurs.[12] Metabolites associated with chronic swelling and fibrotic joint changes are also reduced. From open wounds to chronic tendinitis, all phases of wound healing, except the initial inflammatory stage, benefit from the various forms of heat.

Dependent on the acuity of the wound or soft tissue condition, mild, moderate, or vigorous dosages of heat should be considered.

The connective tissue response involves an improvement in the properties of collagen and the extensibility of tissue when combined with passive or active mobilization and engagement in occupation. Joint stiffness is reduced and range of motion may be improved. A moderate to vigorous dose of heat should be considered.

Therapeutic dosages used clinically include moderate to vigorous forms of heat. Clinical interventions should be able to provide the desired dosage based on temperature selection and conduction factors.

Indications

Many musculoskeletal conditions commonly seen by clinicians benefit from SHAs. Heat can be used to decrease pain and stiffness, improve range of motion and tendon excursion, improve viscosity of synovia, and to promote healing and relaxation. Conditions that benefit from heat include:

- stiff joints
- subcutaneous adhesions
- contractures
- chronic arthritis
- subacute and chronic inflammation/cumulative trauma
- trauma/wounds (judiciously used whirlpool or hydrotherapy)
- neuromas
- sympathetic nervous system disorders
- muscle spasms

Evaluation

The intake interview is a crucial element of evaluation and assessment. It is necessary to identify contraindications that may preclude the use of SHAs. Considerations include:

- past medical history
- pregnancy
- skin condition: color, temperature, sensitivity, dryness, and overall integrity
- medications

Precautions

The OT must take the necessary precautions to assure that the heat treatment is a safe adjunct to the therapeutic program. Increased edema is one drawback of heat application, and positioning and mobilization techniques must be considered to counteract any adverse effects. The therapist should be cautious when treating patients with other associated conditions, such as diminished sensation and compromised circulation. The clinician should monitor the patient's response to the heat agent at all times. Subjective comments related to any negative effects should be immediately addressed. Overt physiological signs must be monitored as well. This includes general skin color and respiratory status. Local signs related to the effects of heat overexposure, such as petechiae and blistering, must also be observed.

Contraindications

Determining whether to use heat as an adjunct to treatment often depends on the intensity of the heat modality under consideration. Sometimes it is necessary to use a mild dose rather than a vigorous dose of heat. Heat should not be used with those patients who have appreciable circulatory impairment.

In occupational therapy, heat is typically used for its local effects. Nevertheless, systemic effects of heat occur from a localized application of heat. Heat is dissipated from local tissue through circulating blood. In individuals with circulatory impairment, the body is unable to efficiently rid itself of heat as readily as those who are healthy. Increased heart rate may result from the systemic effects as well. SHAs should not be used with the following conditions:

- impaired sensation (superficial, skin graft, or scar)
- tumors/cancer
- acute inflammation, including acute edema
- deep vein thrombophlebitis
- pregnancy (the systemic effects of circulating blood on a fetus are unclear)
- bleeding tendencies
- infection
- primary repair of tendon or ligament
- advanced cardiac disease
- semicomatose or impaired mental status
- rheumatoid arthritis (vigorous dosages of heat may facilitate proteins that act as catalysts to increase enzyme activity, exacerbating joint inflammation. [16]

Modality Selection

Modality selection will depend on the objective of superficial heat use, the location and surface area of the involved structure, the desired dosage/tissue temperature, and the desired depth of penetration. Other considerations include: whether moist or dry heat is desired, positioning of the extremity in a (non) dependent or intermittently dependent position, and whether active or passive patient participation is desired. Consideration of whether the condition being treated is acute, subacute, or chronic is also necessary. If depths greater than one centimeter are desired, ultrasound may be indicated.[17] The effect that the SHA will have upon tissue will depend on the temperature of the application site and the type of modality used. [4,5]

Clinical Applications—Convection

Whirlpool Bath/Hydrotherapy

Whirlpool bath or hydrotherapy can be used when a mild, moderate or vigorous dosage of moist heat is desired. *Mosby's Medical, Nursing and Allied Health Dictionary* defines a whirlpool bath as the immersion of a body part in a tank of water agitated by a jet of equal water and air via an electric turbine.[18] One of the properties of water is buoyancy, which helps in producing a gravity-eliminated environment. This environment can be therapeutic for graded active mobilization of an affected body part such as a patient with a wrist fracture which has been immobilized for several weeks.

An advantage to the use of whirlpool bath is that the therapist is able to see and have immediate access to the body part being treated. Water temperature can be controlled and set to the desired temperature. Agitation of the water can be controlled and acts as soft tissue massage and/or a resistance for exercise. If wounds or excessive skin dryness are present, whirlpool bath can be used for cleaning and debridement, which further aids in the healing process. Whirlpool bath is considered an active SHA because the patient can participate in a variety of active movements while in the whirlpool.

A disadvantage in using whirlpool bath is the dependent position in which the extremity being treated is placed. If edema is a concern, the extremity being maintained below the heart may not be desirable. To counteract this, the patient should be instructed to intermittently dry off the body part, such as the hand, and raise it overhead. If feasible, this should be complemented by pumping (fisting) the hand several times in succession. Another disadvantage to utilizing whirlpool is the time required for set up and cleaning, which may be time consuming in busy clinics.

In conclusion, whirlpool baths are an effective modality to use with open wounds, status post fractures (where stiffness and excessive skin dryness is present), inflammatory conditions, peripheral vascular disease and peripheral nerve injuries. The general instructions for use are as follows:

· Therapeutic water temperature of 100-104° F for heating, or 90-100° F for open wounds.[12]
· If the patient does have open wounds, proper disinfecting measures must be taken.
· Optimal length of treatment is approximately 20 minutes (Figure 5-1).

Fluidotherapy

Fluidotherapy can be used as a mild, moderate, or vigorous dosage of dry heat. Analgesic effects can be obtained with lower temperatures and other physiological effects are achieved at higher temperatures. This SHA uses fine particles suspended in a hot air stream to heat the extremity.[5] The fine particles are made of the cellulose from ground up corn husks. The temperature of the circulating air is controlled by a thermostat on the machine. This type of treatment can be used on the distal extremities, primarily the hands and feet (Figure 5-2).

The advantage of using fluidotherapy is the ease of implementation. The machines can be purchased with either single or dual accessibility features which allows the therapist access to the patient's extremity while in the unit, allowing for passive range of motion, joint mobilization, and manipulation. The accessibility feature also allows the treatment of up to two patients at a time. The force of the air and particles circulating within the machine can be graded via the blower speed. The force of the blower speed allows for mobilization to take place during the treatment process. Many therapists use fluidotherapy for the desensitization effects that it provides with abnormally hypersensitive areas.

The disadvantage of fluidotherapy is primarily that the extremity is maintained in the dependent position. The clinician must be prudent in using this modality, particularly if edema is a concern. If edema is a concern, fluidotherapy should be used as an

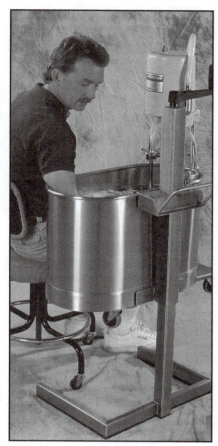

Figure 5-1. Whirlpool. Illustration courtesy of Whitehall Manufacturing, City of Industry, California.

Figure 5-2. Fluidotherapy.

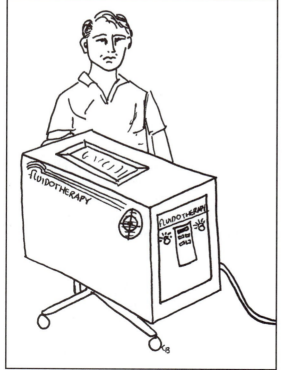

Figure 5-3. SHAs: Hot packs. Illustration by Kim Bartlett. Used with permission.

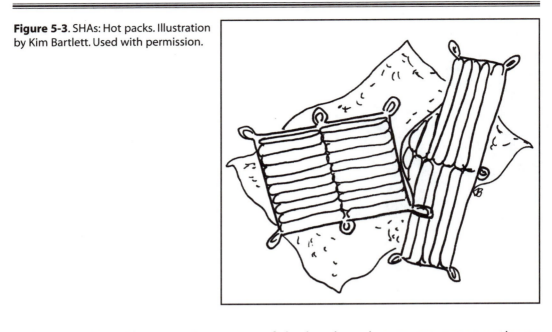

active modality with a pumping action of the hand used to counteract any adverse effects of the heat dosage. A second issue relates to housekeeping duties. If a high volume of patients are treated throughout the day, particles from the machine often end up on the floor.

The first step in using fluidotherapy is to pre-heat the unit to 105-118° F. The blower speed should be set, which provides the desired air and particle flow within the machine. The body part being treated should be clean and free from jewelry. If any open wounds are present, the therapist needs to make sure they are adequately covered before treatment begins. The length of treatment is typically set for approximately 20 minutes.

Clinical Applications—Conduction

Hot Packs

Hot or hydrocollator packs are typically used to provide moderate and vigorous doses of moist heat. Although hot packs come in a variety of sizes, this SHA effectively heats larger areas of the body and adequately covers contoured areas of the body, such as the shoulder. The temperature of the hot pack is typically 104-113° F if stored in water at a desired temperature of 170° F. Hot packs are cooler than water because of the properties that make up the various materials of this heat agent (Figure 5-3).

Hot packs are generally easy to use and require minimal maintenance. Provided they are adequately padded, they are safer than other forms of superficial heat because they become cooler as the treatment progresses. The hot pack is also easy to remove, thereby decreasing the risk of the patient being burned. Hot packs are beneficial in helping to reduce pain and muscle spasms and to improve connective tissue extensibility.[17]

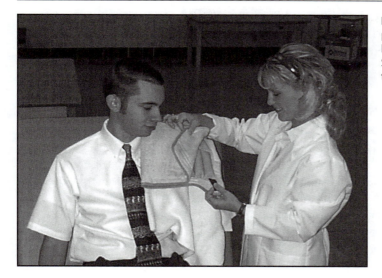

Figure 5-4. Application of hot pack. Treated area should always be padded to prevent burning. Skin condition should be monitored.

Although hot packs are considered a passive treatment, a positional sustained stretch of the tissue being treated can be accomplished during the heating process (Figure 5-4).

A disadvantage to using hot packs is that the larger size hot packs can be heavy and contraindicated if too uncomfortable for the patient. Additionally, the area being treated is covered, making it difficult for the therapist to monitor the patient's skin integrity.[15-19] The general instructions for use are as follows:

- The hot pack is wrapped in several layers of cloth toweling and/or commercial hot pack covers to prevent burns.
- Be aware that pressure from positioning will cause conductive heating. To decrease conduction, reposition body part and add additional toweling. To improve conduction, further secure hot pack with theraband or toweling over the body part being treated, eg, shoulder.
- Treatment length is approximately 20 minutes.
- Allow hot pack to reheat for at least 30 minutes before using it again.

Contrast Bath

Contrast baths provide mild to moderate heat dosages. This SHA is often used with conditions involving impaired blood flow, edema and subacute/chronic inflammation. Contrast baths produce alternating vasodilation and vasoconstriction, which improves peripheral blood flow, aids in healing while controlling edema, and reduces pain and stiffness.[4] Contrast baths are often performed in the patient's own home (home program or home health care) to decrease or control symptoms.

Contrast bath involves alternating the affected extremity between warm and cold water. This can be accomplished by filling two containers with water, one with warm water between 100-110° F and one with cold tap water, typically at a temperature between 50-70° F. Although various protocols exist, the general guidelines are to have the patient immerse the part being treated in warm water for 10 minutes. After the 10 minutes in warm water, the patient should place the body part in cold water for 1 minute. The patient then returns to warm water for 4 minutes and then cold water for 1 minute. This 4:1 cycle is completed two additional times. When a contrast bath is used as a SHA, the patient should end the treatment in 4 minutes of warm water, providing 30 minutes of total treatment.[4]

Warm Water Soak

Warm water soaks can be used when mild or moderate dosages of heat are indicated. This type of SHA provides circumferential heat to the fingers and allows the patient to mobilize the hand and fingers to improve range of motion and decrease subacute and chronic edema. This form of hydrotherapy is ideal for a home program. The temperature is typically initiated at 99-110° F. The water is in a container that the person's extremity can fit into. A 15-20 minute immersion is generally indicated. If edema is a concern, the patient may be instructed in controlling the potential edema by actively moving the part being treated while in the dependent position, or to intermittently elevate the extremity above her heart.

Paraffin Bath

The paraffin bath provides moderate to vigorous dosages of heat. This SHA can provide a high degree of localized heat to the smaller joints. It is used primarily to decrease stiffness and improve range of motion. It also offers pain control. Healed amputations, arthritis, and strains/sprains are just a few conditions that benefit from paraffin.

The paraffin bath must be accompanied by a thermostat to ensure patient safety. The heated storage unit contains a mixture of paraffin and mineral oil. The temperature is typically between 118-135° F.[2] Paraffin has a lower specific heat than water so the paraffin will feel cooler to the patient than water at the same temperature.[19] Mineral oil contained in the paraffin lowers the melting point and allows for ease of removal of the paraffin from the body part.

A primary advantage of paraffin is that it allows for an even distribution of heat to the treatment surface, which is effective in reducing stiffness and pain. This form of heat also reduces the viscosity of the synovia, reducing the stiffness associated with arthritis. When using paraffin with rheumatoid arthritis, it is imperative that one refrain from administering a vigorous heat dosage. The temperature of the paraffin should be maintained at the lower range. The provision of paraffin is easy, efficient, and rather inexpensive. Passive stretching of joints can be accomplished with an elastic-type wrap. This form of treatment can be used in conjunction with the paraffin to maximize the benefits of mobilizing connective tissue.

The disadvantage of this SHA is that it cannot be easily used on all body parts. Although paraffin does gradually cool after being applied, there is no mechanism to control the temperature of the paraffin once it is applied to the skin. Because it is difficult to regulate the temperature, the risk of burns is substantially higher than other forms of heat. Paraffin should not be used with open wounds or over joints which are acutely inflamed. Paraffin maintains a therapeutic temperature for about 20 minutes.[15] Paraffin can be applied in a variety of ways, including wrap/gloving, immersion,dip, brush and pouring methods.

Wrap/Gloving Technique: This method may be the most popular method of paraffin application by the occupational therapist. The therapist should first observe the temperature of the paraffin unit's thermometer for safety, demonstrate the technique,

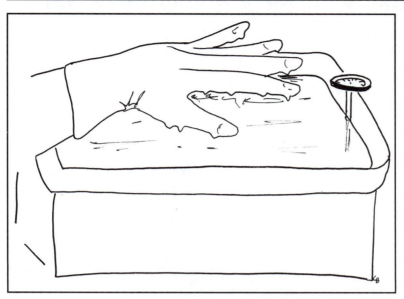

Figure 5-5. Paraffin. Illustration by Kim Bartlett. Used with permission.

and then ask the patient to slowly place her fingertips into the paraffin. The patient is then instructed to immerse the part into the bath while avoiding contact with the bottom and the sides of the paraffin unit. Once this first dip is completed, the patient is instructed to immediately remove the extremity and allow it to air dry for a few seconds prior to immersing once again. The dip process, referred to as "gloving," is repeated approximately 10 times depending on the patient's tolerance to the heat. The therapist then wraps the part in a large plastic bag and a cloth towel is wrapped around to serve as an insulating layer retaining the heat. Typical treatment time lasts 20 minutes. At the conclusion of treatment, the paraffin should be removed and discarded (Figure 5-5).

Immersion Technique: At an elevated therapeutic temperature of 125-135° F, this technique will provide a vigorous dosage of heat. The patient immerses and leaves her hand in the paraffin bath for approximately 10-20 minutes.

Dip Immersion Technique: Depending on the therapeutic temperature of the paraffin, this will provide a moderate or vigorous dosage of heat. This involves the gloving method noted earlier. Instead of wrapping the body part as the final step, the area being treated remains within the paraffin bath (Figure 5-6).

Brush Technique: This process involves using a paint brush and brushing eight to 10 coats of paraffin onto an area that cannot be dipped, such as the lateral epicondyle at the elbow area. The treated area is wrapped with towels for approximately 20 minutes. A moderate dosage of heat can be obtained.

Pouring Technique: This process can be used for the same reasons that brushing may be used. It may also be indicated when treating the hand, especially if the patient is unable immerse her hand into the bath.

Figure 5-6. Paraffin application. Following the dipping procedure, the extremity will be wrapped in the plastic bag and then the towel. Skin condition should be monitored. Temperature of the paraffin should be checked before application.

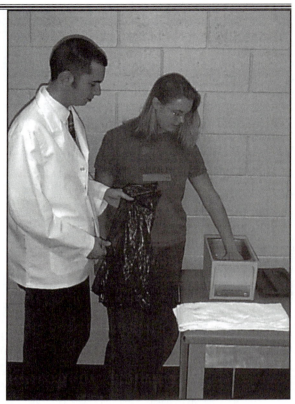

Case Study

Doug is a 33 y/o father of three young children. He incurred a traumatic injury to his right dominant hand while working at a local hospital within the maintenance department. He sustained musculoskeletal, vascular, and nervous tissue injuries, in addition to amputation of his third and fourth distal phalanges. One week following surgery, Doug was referred to occupational therapy for wound management and dressing, range of motion as tolerated, and splinting.

Initially, treatment consisted of whirlpool at a tepid temperature of approximately 90° F. Mild agitation was allowed. This process was favorable to cleaning the hand and wounds and also facilitated the healing process. Within the subacute stage of healing, approximately 3 1/2 weeks postsurgery, the wounds closed and greater range of motion was warranted. Whirlpool continued to be the modality of choice due to the minimal edema that was present. The physiological effects of mild heat coupled with the intermittent ability of countering the effects of edema with elevation and active range of motion were the determinants for modality selection at this phase. Immediately following SHAs application, therapeutic occupations were implemented. During the subacute stage, skin integrity continued to improve, edema was considerably decreased, and all aspects of the musculoskeletal injuries were healed. Fluidotherapy was now the SHA of choice, providing moderate to vigorous doses of heat while allowing Doug to actively mobilize his hand and fingers during treatment. He also benefited from the desensitization effects of the modality which normalized his hyperesthesia. The dependent position of the extremity during the 20 minute treatment was no longer a concern. Finally, as Doug participated in functional job simulated activity, he recognized the positive thermal benefits of heat to the persistent stiffness that he was experiencing. Paraffin was then used prior to his engagement in therapeutic occupation. The thermal effects of paraffin were complemented by a sustained passive composite finger flexion stretch that was obtained with Coban wrap as a part of treatment. SHAs allowed Doug to maximize his participation and performance in treatment and he quickly returned to his position within the maintenance department without restrictions. Doug's scenario demonstrates how occupational therapy intervention (from the most acute stages to return to work) can provide remedial and compensatory treatment such that an individual can fully return to his or her occupational roles.

Summary

Purposeful occupation is what occupational therapists value. It is our treatment medium. Participation in therapeutic occupation improves the volition of a person and facilitates wellness, adaptation, and engagement in life. As clinicians, we have the challenge of appropriately integrating SHAs into practice. The use of SHAs in the treatment process is a service need and expectation of patients, physicians, and payers. With certain patients, SHAs can serve as an important adjunct to treatment. Clinicians must be competent and proficient with SHA usage to safely and effectively use them in clinical practice. SHAs facilitate tissue healing and extensibility, and decrease pain by impacting the neurovascular, neuromuscular, and metabolic processes of the body. For some patients, SHAs can prepare patients for their participation in therapeutic occupation.

References

1. Post R, Lee S, Syen D. Physical agent modalities. In: Trombly C, ed. *Occupational Therapy for Physical Dysfunction*. 4th ed. Baltimore, Md: Williams & Wilkins; 1995:659-661.

2. Cannon N, Mullins PT. Modalities in upper extremity rehabilitation. In: Malick M, Kasch M, eds. *Manual on Management of Specific Hand Problems, Series 1*. Pittsburgh, Pa: American Rehabilitation Educational Network; 1984:72-75.

3. Kaul MP. Superficial heat and cold. *The Physician and Sportsmedicine*. 1994;22:65-74.

4. Lehmann JF, DeLateur BJ. Therapeutic heat. In: *Therapeutic Heat and Cold*. 4th ed. Baltimore, Md: Williams & Wilkins; 1990;417-457:590-632.

5. Borrell RM, Parker R, Henley EJ, Masley D, Repinecz M. Comparison of in vivo temperatures produced by hydrotherapy, paraffin wax treatment, and fluidotherapy. *Physical Therapy*. 1980;60:1273-1276.

6. Greenburg RS. The effects of hot packs and exercise on local blood flow. *Physical Therapy*. 1972;52:273-279.

7. Lehmann J. *Therapeutic Heat and Cold*. 3rd ed. Baltimore, MD: Williams and Wilkins; 1982:65.

8. Norkin C, Levangie P. *Joint Structure and Function: A Comprehensive Analysis*. 2nd ed. Philadelphia, Pa: FA Davis; 1992:79-81.

9. Lehmann J, Warren G, Scham S. Therapeutic heat and cold. *Clinical Orthopedics and Related Research*. 1974;99:207-245.

10. Sekins KM, Lehmann JF, Esselman P, et al. Local muscle blood flow and temperature responses to 915 MHz diathermy as simultaneously measured and numerically predicted. *Archives of Physical Medicine and Rehabilitation*. 1984;65:1-7.

11. Hoban C. *Therapeutic heat*. One day presentation at the Michigan Occupational Therapy Association fall conference. October 1, 1993.

12. Hayes KW. *Manual for Physical Agents*. 4th ed. Norwalk, CT: Appleton & Lange; 1993.

13. Moritz A, Henrique F. Studies of thermal injury, Part II: The relative importance of time and surface temperature in the causation of cutaneous burns. *American Journal of Pathology*. 1947;23:695-720.

14. DeJong R, Hershey W, Wagman I. Nerve conduction velocity during hypothermia in man. *Anesthesiology*. 1966;27:805-810.

15. Michlovitz SL. Biophysical principles of heating and superficial heat agents. In: Michlovitz SL, Wolf SL. *Thermal Agents in Rehabilitation*. 1st ed. Philadelphia, Pa: FA Davis; 1986:99-118.

16. Schmidt KL. Heat, cold and inflammation. *Rheumatology*. 1979;38:391-404.

17. Michlovitz SL. Biophysical principles of heating and superficial heat agents. In:Michlovitz SL. *Thermal Agents in Rehabilitation*. 2nd ed. Philadelphia, Pa: F.A. Davis; 1990:88-108.

18. *Mosby's Medical, Nursing, and Allied Health Dictionary*. St. Louis, MO: Mosby Year-book, Inc; 1994.

Bibliography

Hecox B. Terminology. In: Hecox B, Mehreteab T, Weisberg J, eds. *Physical Agents: A Comprehensive Text for Physical Therapists*. Norwalk, CT: Appleton & Lange; 1994: 59-60.

Chapter Six

Therapeutic Ultrasound & Phonophoresis

Learning Objectives

1. Discuss the theory and principles of therapeutic ultrasound.
2. Discuss the biophysiological changes which occur with ultrasound.
3. Discuss the different parameters used in therapeutic ultrasound.
4. Discuss the clinical applications for the use of therapeutic ultrasound.

Terminology

Beam Nonuniformity Ratio	Phonophoresis
Cavitation	Piezoelectric Effect
Duty Cycle	Pulsed
Frequency	Reverse Piezoelectric Effect
Intensity	Shear Wave
Nonthermal Effect	Thermal Effect

Ultrasound is considered a deep heat modality which can be used as an adjunct to facilitate occupational performance during occupational therapy treatment. By definition, ultrasound is acoustic energy which is inaudible by the human ear, due to a frequency greater than 20 kilohertz (kHz). The frequency band for medical ultrasound is 800,000 to 3,000,000 Hz (0.8 to 3 MHz). With the impetus of managed care to rehabilitate patients faster, cheaper, and more effectively, occupational therapists have been advancing their knowledge and practice base using technologies and applications to facilitate the healing process and speed recovery. Historically, occupational therapists have employed paraffin or hot packs to "heat" selected tissues. Therapeutic ultrasound is an additional method which can be a beneficial adjunct to the occupational therapy process.

Classification

Therapeutic ultrasound is a thermal modality which can be used to heat structures superficially (0-1cm), or at greater depths (up to 5 cm). The most common frequency in use for therapeutic ultrasound is 1 MHz (1 million cycles/second), while newer units provide an additional setting of 3 MHz (Figure 6-1).

Therapeutic ultrasound produces tissue change through both a thermal and non-thermal effect and can be used as an adjunct to occupational performance. Thermal agents have two primary classifications: superficial and deep. Superficial thermal agents elevate tissue temperature to a depth of approximately 1 cm. Therapeutic ultrasound is considered a deep-heating thermal agent capable of elevating tissue temperatures to a depth of 5 cm or more.[1] A frequency of 1 MHz will provide deeper penetration than 3 MHz.

Therapeutic ultrasound has two primary purposes: to elevate tissue temperature and to provide nonthermal secondary cellular effects. In order to safely and effectively use ultrasound in the treatment process, it is necessary to understand its history, principles, effects, indications, and contraindications.

History

Ultrasound consists of an acoustic energy and has been used in medicine for diagnosis and tissue destruction, and in physical medicine and rehabilitation to help restore and heal soft tissues. In 1880, Pierre and Jacques Curies discovered that certain crystals, such as quartz, lithium sulfate, and zinc oxide, generated an electrical charge when mechanically compressed. The Curies discovered that the crystals produce positive and negative electrical charges when they expand and contract, known as the piezoelectric effect. An indirect or reverse piezoelectric effect is the contraction or expansion of a crystal which occurs in response to electrical voltage being applied. The reverse piezoelectric effect is the production of mechanical energy secondary to the application of an electrical charge across the crystal. The polarity changes cause the crystal to oscillate and deform in response to the electrical current. Ultrasound uses the reverse piezoelectric effect to produce the high-frequency sound waves. The application of alternating current makes the crystal vibrate at the frequency of the electrical oscillation, generating a variety of frequencies.[2]

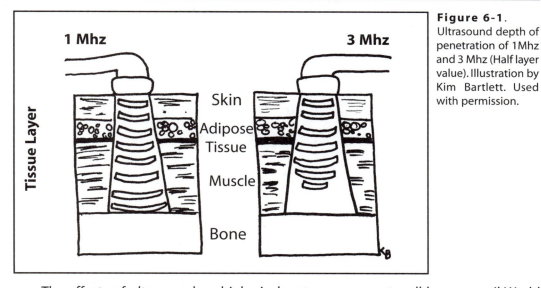

Figure 6-1.
Ultrasound depth of penetration of 1Mhz and 3 Mhz (Half layer value). Illustration by Kim Bartlett. Used with permission.

The effects of ultrasound on biological systems were not well known until World War I. During this period of technological advances, researchers were attempting to devise methods for detecting submarines which were sinking Allied shipping vessels. When researchers were developing devices to locate submarines undersea, they found that a piezoelectric transducer emitted ultrasonic waves into the ocean following excitation. Surprisingly, the amplitude of the acoustic waves was at times strong enough to kill marine animals and small fish. Researchers continued to explore the biologic effects on tissues exposed to these high-frequency sound waves during the 1930s and 1940s, with the application of ultrasound for medical treatment occurring in Germany and then in the United States.[3,4]

Ultrasound Equipment

The basis for current ultrasound equipment was derived from the Curies' work on crystal oscillation and voltage polarization. The standard ultrasound unit consists of a power supply, oscillator circuit, transformer, coaxial cable transducer and ultrasound applicator. Most often, therapeutic ultrasound units have a generator which uses common house current (alternating current) as a power source, and converts this electrical energy into ultrasonic energy. With therapeutic ultrasound machines, the crystal is located inside the applicator, which is called a transducer. The crystal consists of natural quartz or a synthetic material that vibrates by contracting and expanding in response to alternating current. Each crystal has a unique, naturally occurring vibration frequency to which the electronics of the ultrasound unit are matched (Figure 6-2). Because of this, ultrasound transducers are not interchangeable between units. Some of the current manufacturers, however, have solved this problem and are producing interchangeable sound heads. The vibration of the crystal generates pressure waves which affect the tissue. The crystal deforms in response to the changes in the direction of the flow of the current and is proportional to the amount of voltage applied to the crystal. In therapeutic ultrasound, these pressure waves are transmitted to a small volume of tissue which cause the molecules to vibrate. Ultrasound travels poorly through air so a lubricant is used that allows the energy to be dispersed into the tissue (Figure 6-3).

Transmission relative to water (%)	Media/products that transmit ultrasound well:
97%	Lidex gel, fluocinonide 0.05%
97%	Thera-Gesic cream, methyl salicylate 15%
97%	Mineral oil
96%	US gel
90%	US lotion
88%	Betamethasone 0.05% in US gel
	Media/products that transmit US poorly:
36%	Diprolene ointment, betamethasone 0.05%
29%	Hydrocortisone (HC) powder 1% in US gel
7%	HC powder 10% in US gel
	Media/product with zero transmissivity:
0%	Cortil ointment, HC 1%
0%	Eucerin cream
0%	HC cream 1%
0%	HC cream 10%
0%	HC cream 10%, mixed with equal weight US gel
0%	Myoglex cream, trolamine salicylate 10%
0%	Triamcinolone acetonide cream 0.1%
0%	Velva HC cream 10%
0%	Velva HC cream 10% with equal weight US gel
0%	White petrolatum
	Other
68%	Chempad-L
98%	Polyethylene wrap

Figure 6-2. Ultrasound transmission by phonophoresis according to media. Adapted from Cameron MH, Monroe LG. Relative transmission of ultrasound by media customarily used for phonophoresis. *Physical Therapy*. 1992; 72(2):145.

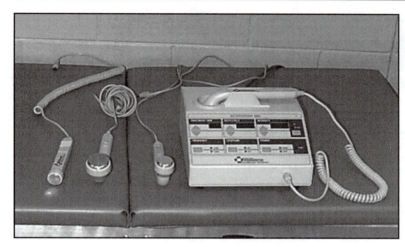

Figure 6-3. Ultrasound equipment. Note the three different size sound heads: 10 cm, 5 cm, and 2 cm.

Physical Principles

The sound waves created by the ultrasound unit can be visualized as being similar to waves in a pond created when a stone is tossed into the middle. The peak and trough of the sound waves mirror the phases of compression and rarefaction of the crystal. In ultrasound equipment, when alternating current is applied to the crystal, it expands and contracts, causing the acoustical or sound waves. Due to the rapid generation of the sound waves, molecules in the wave's path are pushed back and forth by the alternating phases of successive waves until the wave runs out of energy. This type of wave, which moves in one direction, compressing and decompressing the molecules in its way, is known as a longitudinal wave.

Ultrasound can be transmitted, absorbed, reflected, and refracted depending on the type of tissue that the energy affects, and the angle of the wave. The rate at which the sound wave travels is dependent, in part, on the density of the molecules of the specific tissue. There is an inverse relationship between absorption and penetration. If the tissue molecules are widely dispersed, there is a low absorption of the sound energy, and the depth of penetration is greater. If the molecules of the tissue are close together or compressed, the rate at which the sound will travel will be less as the energy is absorbed because the molecules resist compression.

When the particle movement is at right angles to the propagation of the wave, a shear or transverse wave is created. This occurs in solid substances. Liquid substances, which have weaker intramolecular bonds, are less able to transmit the shear wave. Clinically, shear waves occur when a pressure wave reaches a bone, with the wave being generated along the periosteum. This shear wave may cause heating of the outer covering of the bone.[5]

Each tissue in the body has a different density, and each will transmit and absorb ultrasound according to its unique acoustical properties. Researchers have identified the acoustic absorption coefficient of various body tissues. Body fluids, such as blood and water, have the lowest impedance and acoustic absorption coefficient. Conversely, bone has the highest impedance and acoustic absorption coefficient, making it a good absorber of ultrasound energy.[6,7] It is through understanding of the tissue healing process and appreciating the acoustic absorption coefficient of body tissues with the tissue response, that therapeutic ultrasound becomes an important adjunct to the treatment process (Table 6-1).

Table 6-1. Acoustic Impedance Level	
Tissue Type	**Impedance** (kg/m@sec x 10(6))
Fat	1.38
Water	1.5
Blood	1.61
Muscle	1.7
Bone	7.8

Overview of Wound Healing

The body's response to an injury occurs in a fairly consistent pattern, which is an attempt to return the tissue to its normal state. Occupational therapists should have a clear understanding of wound healing to appreciate the significance and impact of physical agents, and particularly therapeutic ultrasound, on the healing process.

Wound healing can be considered a process of essentially three events that occur in response to an injury: inflammation, tissue repair, and remodeling. The phases of wound healing and the biologic repair process are the same for all wounds, although the sequence of repair and the speed of the process will vary depending on the type of wound.

Inflammation, the initial stage of injury, is a vascular, hemostatic, cellular, and immune response to the initial insult. It is the body's attempt to dispose of foreign material and dead tissue, and is characterized by skin color change, elevated temperature (heat), swelling (turgor), increased sensation (usually pain), and a concurrent loss of function. The process of inflammation lasts approximately 3 to 7 days, with acute inflammation occurring at the initial onset of the injury and disrupting normal tissue physiology.

The second phase of healing—tissue repair—is considered the proliferative phase, involving fibroplasia and wound contraction. Fibroplasia is the process where the body lays down a collagen matrix known as granulation tissue, which is structurally and functionally different than the tissue it replaces. Granulation tissue does not differentiate into the respective tissue that it is replacing, such as nerves, muscles, and tendons. Wound contraction is the process of pulling the wound edges together in an attempt to close the wound. Myofibroblasts migrate to the wound skin margin and pull the epidermal layer inward. This is described as a "picture frame" effect.

The final phase of wound healing, remodeling, may last for many years and is characterized by collagen lysis, a process affecting the organization of the collagen fibers into fibers that are more elastic, smoother, and stronger. It is during the process of scar formation that therapists attempt to manipulate the alignment of the collagen fibers based on tension theory; the internal and external stresses that affect the wound.

During this stage of recovery, the use of deeper, penetrating ultrasound can be used to heat the fibers, with the therapist using passive, active, or positional stretch to stress and elongate the tissue.

It is important to emphasize that the phases of wound healing do not occur in isolation to each other but are overlapping and dynamic. Age; nutrition; metabolic disorders; peripheral vascular disease; the presence of diabetes; and medications such as corticosteroids, NSAIDs, and others may negatively affect the healing process. Physical agents, such as ultrasound, can be used to facilitate or accelerate the healing process, as well as to control undesirable effects of the injury. Thermal agents such as ultrasound and physical technologies in general should never be used in isolation of other treatment techniques or intervention, but used to facilitate an individual's occupational performance.

Energy Distribution

The therapeutic effect of tissue heating is due to the distribution of energy in the ultrasound field. The width or spread of the ultrasound is affected by the frequency and size of the crystal. The larger the sound head or transducer (and therefore the crystal), the greater the divergence of the field. There is variation of the energy within the sound wave caused by a number of mechanisms, with peaks and troughs of the sound wave in the near field and the far field.

The spatial peak intensity (SPI) is the maximum intensity appearing at any point in the beam. The spatial average intensity (SAI) is the average intensity over the area of the beam of energy. The intensity is higher in some areas of the ultrasound beam than others. The relationship between the SPI and the SAI is called the beam nonuniformity ratio (BNR) and is reported by the manufacturer for each ultrasound machine.[8,9] These higher intensity areas within the ultrasound beam are a primary cause for the "hot spots" which may occur during application, and are prevented, in part, by keeping the sound head moving throughout the treatment.

Intensity describes the strength of the acoustic energy at the site of application. Intensity is determined by measuring the acoustic power (Watts) of the applicator and dividing it by the effective radiating area (ERA) (sq. cm) of the transducer (W/cm^2). The intensity is the most significant factor in determining a tissue response. As a general rule, the greater the intensity, the greater the resulting tissue temperature elevation. The intensity of an ultrasound unit should always be decreased if the patient experiences discomfort at any time. Complaints of an "ache" or "shooting" or "stabbing" pain are indications that the intensity should be decreased or the sound head should be moved more rapidly.[10]

The duty cycle is used to determine the overall amount of acoustic energy that a patient receives. This cycle also is a vital factor in determining the tissue response to the sound wave. The duty cycle is frequently seen as a percentage or ratio of the on-time of the pulse, the duration the unit is on to the pulse period. A 50% duty cycle would provide twice as much acoustic energy as a 25% duty cycle since the on-time is twice as long. The temporal peak intensity is the maximum intensity of the sound wave during the on phase of pulsed ultrasound. The temporal average intensity is the intensity average over a given time span, which includes both on- and off- time.[11] The choice of continuous or pulsed ultrasound is dependent on the pathology, the stage of wound healing, and the amount of area to be treated.[12]

Physiological Effects

Thermal or Continuous-Mode Ultrasound

The physiological effects of tissue heating are the same regardless of how the heat is applied. One of the primary advantages in using therapeutic ultrasound is the ability to target selected treatment sites. Superficial thermal agents can heat tissue to 1 cm, whereas low frequency ultrasound can penetrate selected tissues up to 5 cm. To achieve a thermal effect, intensities of 1.0 to 2.0 W/cm² are used in a continuous mode for between 5 and 8 minutes. When ultrasound is used in a continuous mode for its thermal effect, it is considered a deep-heating modality.

Patients, and some occupational therapists, often think that the ultrasound unit produces heat and sends it to the tissue. In fact, the ultrasound beam does not itself transmit heat. Heat accumulates in the tissue by the conversion of kinetic energy, which is absorbed from the sound wave in continuous-mode or high-intensity ultrasound.

Energy is also absorbed from the ultrasound beam in proportion to the density of the tissue. Protein-dense structures such as scar tissue, capsules, ligaments, tendons, and bones accumulate heat readily and selectively absorb the ultrasound energy. Because of the propensity of protein dense structures to absorb the ultrasound, therapists can selectively heat dense or deep lying tissues.[13-15] Due to the extensive capillary network, muscles lose heat more quickly than the more dense structures.

Ultrasound has the potential to cause two types of cavitation, stable and unstable. Cavitation is the formation and collapse of gas or vapor filled cavities in liquids, and occurs in relation to the compression and rarefaction cycles of the ultrasound. Cavitation causes an expansion and compression of these small gas bubbles which may be present in blood or tissue fluids located in the ultrasound beam's path. Cavitation occurs as a result of the pressure changes caused by the sound wave generation.

Thermal effects of tissue heating can also occur due to cavitation. Micron sized gas bubbles are present in the body fluids within the sound wave. With the application of higher intensity, these bubbles can reach a critical size and collapse, causing unstable cavitation. In unstable cavitation, energy is released into the surrounding tissue, causing an increase in temperature and damage to the tissue, blood cells, and other tissue located within the sound wave (Figure 6-4). Unstable cavitation occurs more frequently with 1 MHz ultrasound than with 3 MHz ultrasound, and can be avoided by using higher frequencies and avoiding the development of hot spots caused by the therapist failing to move the sound head consistently.

A number of physiological effects occur in tissue when thermal modalities, including thermal ultrasound, are used.

> **Physiologic changes which occur with tissue heating include:**
> - increased metabolic rates of tissue
> - increased blood flow and tissue permeability
> - increased viscoelasticity of connective tissue
> - elevation of pain thresholds
> - increased enzymatic reactivity, stimulating the immune system

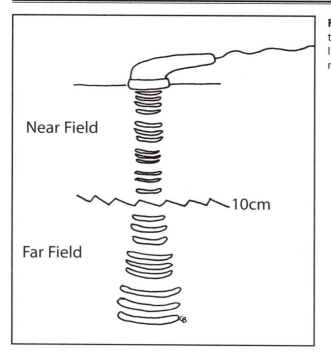

Figure 6-4. Transmission of Ultrasound through large homogeneous tissue. Illustration by Kim Bartlett. Used with permission.

Clinically, thermal ultrasound is used to increase joint range of motion, facilitate tissue healing, decrease muscle spasm, decrease pain, and decrease chronic inflammatory process.[16-19] Because of the ability to selectively set the parameters for ultrasound, occupational therapists can effectively target specific tissues and structures to take advantage of the thermal effects of ultrasound in the healing process.

Nonthermal or Mechanical Ultrasound

When the heating effects of ultrasound are decreased by applying very low-intensity ultrasound or by pulsing it, cellular or mechanical changes occur. The physiologic effects of nonthermal ultrasound are often more significant to the therapist than thermal ultrasound in manipulating the wound healing process. Nonthermal ultrasound causes a destabilization of the cell membrane, causing increased cellular permeability, diffusion, and a cascade of second order effects. Use of pulsed or nonthermal ultrasound has been clinically shown to facilitate tissue repair.[20]

The nonthermal effects of pulsed ultrasound occur at the cell membrane due to mechanical vibrations causing cavitation, acoustic streaming, and micro-massage. The radiation force which occurs during the compression phase of pulsed ultrasound deforms the cell membrane, massaging the cell. Stable cavitation also occurs, with the gas bubbles expanding and contracting in relation to the compression and rarefaction phases of the sound wave.[21] This stable cavitation causes eddy currents in the fluid surrounding the vibrating bubbles, exerting a force and stress on nearby cells.

The unidirectional movement of the fluid within the pressure field is known as acoustic streaming and causes structural changes in the cell and an increase in cell permeability.[22,23] The destabilization of the cellular membrane allows the second-order effects of nonthermal ultrasound to occur. Changes in the cell membrane facilitate the diffusion of ions and metabolites such as calcium ions and histamine across the cell.[24] Calcium is a messenger for protein synthesis, while histamine is found in platelets, within mast cells, and granular leukocytes, and are influential in the vascular and cellular events of inflammation. Secondary effects of pulsed ultrasound include an increase of phagocytic activity of macrophages, an increase in the number and motility of fibroblasts with enhanced protein synthesis, increased granular tissue, and angiogensis facilitating wound contraction.[25] Some research has also indicated that low intensity pulsed ultrasound can accelerate fracture healing in tibial and Colles fractures.[26,27] High intensity, thermal ultrasound parameters (higher than 1.5 w/cm^2) could disrupt the bone healing process and should not be used.

Contrary to the popular belief that ultrasound is most effective for its thermal effects, the nonthermal secondary effects of pulsed ultrasound have a great impact on the wound healing process. Ultrasound can facilitate resolution of the inflammatory phase of healing, and stimulate fibroblastic activity and maturation. In contrast, high-intensity ultrasound (1 MHz, 1.5 w/cm^2) can disrupt tissue repair and aggravate symptoms during the acute phase of healing.[26-28]

In general, the effects of nonthermal ultrasound on tissue healing occur with short treatment durations and lower parameters of 0.1 and 0.2 W/cm^2 doses, pulsed at a 20% duty cycle. As always, a frequency of 1 MHz will provide deeper penetration (up to 5 cm) than 3 MHz. To best facilitate tissue repair, treatment sessions should be repeated every 24 to 48 hours.

Applications and Indications

Ultrasound can be safely and effectively used to treat a variety of clinical conditions seen by the occupational therapist. As with any intervention, a thorough evaluation of the patient is required to identify problems and to set treatment goals. Ultrasound should not be used independently of other treatment approaches, and should be used to impact the healing process. Attention should be paid to the depth and anatomic location of the injury, the area and type of tissue to be treated, and any medical or surgical interventions which have taken place. Clearly identifying the site and depth of the pathology is important because the desired depth of ultrasound penetration will in part determine the frequency. For example, with epicondylitis, the tissue is superficially located, and a frequency of 3 MHz would be more effective in achieving the therapeutic benefits of the ultrasound. When thermal effects are not warranted, for example in a subacute condition or a superficial pathology located near a bony prominence, low intensities should be used.[28]

One of the primary considerations for the therapist is to determine whether to stimulate the healing process through low intensity, pulsed ultrasound, or whether tissue heating is desired through high intensity, constant ultrasound. The initial treatment should usually be of shorter duration than subsequent treatments, and acute conditions should be treated for shorter periods of time than chronic conditions. Smaller areas of tissue also require less treatment time than larger areas, particularly to achieve thermal effects.[29]

Ultrasound may be used before initiating functional activity due to its pain-relieving effects. The sequence of ultrasound use in the treatment process is based, in part, on the identified goals, treatment approach, and desired outcomes determined from the evaluation. Most often, the goal of thermal ultrasound is to increase tissue length. How the tissue is stretched (positional stretch, splinting, functional activities, joint mobilization techniques) is less important than the fact that heated tissues should be stretched

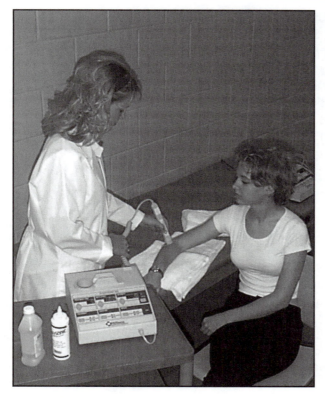

Figure 6-5. Ultrasound application. Note the small sound head to localize the sound wave. Adequate electrode gel is necessary to maintain adequate contact. The sound head should be moved slowly in circles. A 3 MHz frequency is used for superficial tissue.

gently through the pain-free range soon after the application of ultrasound. The targeted tissue stays heated for approximately 8 to 10 minutes, followed by a cool-down period.[30,31]

In general, acute conditions are best treated with lower-intensity dosages of between 0.1 and 0.5 W/cm². With an intensity this low, the patient is unlikely to feel any warmth. Subacute conditions can be treated using a low-intensity dosage of 0.5 to 1.0 W/cm². For chronic conditions or to achieve a thermal change in the tissue, a setting of between 1.0 and 2.0 W/cm² should be used. The patient may experience some degree of warmth but should not report any pain, discomfort, or burning. If this occurs, the intensity should be reduced immediately and the sound head should be moved more quickly. An inadequate amount of ultrasound gel may cause an uncomfortable tingling sensation or vibration. Adding additional gel or applying the ultrasound in water may reduce the patient's discomfort[32-34] (Figure 6-5).

Treatment Frequency and Documentation

Ultrasound is an effective, easy to apply technology. Most often, ultrasound is administered once a day or every other day. It can be safely used as long as there is continued improvement in the patient's condition. As with any treatment intervention, ongoing reassessment of the patients condition, response to intervention, and attainment of goals and outcomes is necessary.

There are no hard and fast answers with regard to the number of treatment sessions using ultrasound. Clinically, many therapists have adhered to a course of 9-12 sessions as long as improvement is noted. The patient's condition is then monitored for approximately 2 weeks. If the condition worsens during that time, an additional series of treatments can be implemented. Some clinical conditions, such as Dupuytren's contractures, may require an extended period of treatment. It should be noted that there are no controlled studies indicating that extended periods of treatment are detrimental, particularly if the patient continues to make progress.

Clear and accurate documentation is necessary to assure continuity between therapists and third party intermediaries. When documenting ultrasound, therapists should note the patient's position, the area being treated, the technique being used (moving sound head, immersion), the frequency (1 MHz or 3 MHz), pulse ratio, intensity, and duration of the treatment. Clearly documenting the sequence of the treatment protocol and the activities and techniques involved, as well as the patient's response to the intervention, is also important.

Precautions and Contraindications

As with any treatment modality, careful observation of the effect of the intervention is important. Therapeutic ultrasound should never be applied over the eye, over the heart, over the pregnant uterus, or over the testes. Due to the possibility of metastasis and increased tumor growth at therapeutic parameters, sonification to malignant tissue should be avoided. Care should also be used when applying ultrasound over areas with decreased circulation or over areas of thrombophlebitis, due to the possibility of clotting or dislodging a thrombus. Growth plates in children should be avoided if possible, particularly higher intensities.[35-37]

Therapists should avoid using a stationary transducer technique due to the increased risk of "hot spots" in the sound field. Patients should not "feel" the ultrasound and should not experience discomfort during the session. If the patient complains of pain, it is usually an indication of periosteal heating. Decreasing the intensity or moving the transducer more quickly should prevent patient discomfort. Patients with surgical metal implants and those with prosthetic joint implants or replacements can safely receive therapeutic ultrasound if appropriate application techniques are followed. There is the possibility of a standing wave developing in metal implants, as the metal reflects approximately 90% of the ultrasound. Plastic is similar to bone in its response to ultrasound, and absorbs a large percentage of the ultrasound. Using the proper application techniques of moving the sound head over the area to be treated and setting the correct treatment parameters is necessary. In general, it is safe to apply ultrasound over implanted materials if proper techniques and precautions are followed.[38-41]

Phonophoresis

Phonophoresis is the use of ultrasound to enhance the delivery of topically applied drugs, most frequently corticosteroids. Phonophoresis has been used clinically with great frequency as therapists attempt to impact the healing process. There have been inconsistencies regarding the effectiveness of phonophoresis in the research because of the variability in outcomes, due in part to the mechanism of delivery. The variability of the treatment parameters: intensity, continuous vs. pulsed, frequency, duration, etc., often conflict.[41-46] It is clear, however, that ultrasound exerts thermal, mechanical, and chemical effects of tissue. The primary factor often neglected or overlooked by clinicians is the type of transmission media utilized.

Transmissivity of ultrasound is directly related to the conducting gel being utilized with wide variability noted. In comparing 19 media, Cameron and Monroe found only six that transmitted at 80% of water or greater, including: plain ultrasound gel (96%), ultrasound lotion (90%), mineral oil (97%), 0.05% betamethasone in ultrasound gel (88%), theragesic cream, 19% methyl salicylate (97%), and Lidex gel, 0.05% fluocinonide (97%). None of the hydrocortisone powders or creams in any percentage transmitted well, and the most commonly used hydrocortisone creams in the clinic— 1% or 10% hydrocortisone in a thick white cream base— did not transmit ultrasound at all, and are ineffective in therapeutic value. Dexamethasone sodium phosphate mixed with a sonic gel has been found to transmit ultrasound more effectively than hydrocortisone acetate and can be formulated by a pharmacist. The thick, white cream base consisting of 10% or 1% hydrocortisone transmits ultrasound poorly and should not be used.

A dressing that seals the area and prevents the escape of moisture should be applied after the treatment. Pretreating the skin with heat, moistening, or shaving the skin should precede application of the phonophoresis. An intensity of 1.5 W/cm^2 should be used for both the thermal and nonthermal effects of the ultrasound with the application of low intensity ultrasound (0.5 W/cm^2) for treating open wounds or acute injuries.[47-49]

Case Study

Jim is a 32 y/o male employed as a production worker on the midnight shift at a small injection molding factory. He lives in a rural town with his wife, a 10-year-old son practicing for the softball team, and two daughters, aged 5 and 7, who are involved in gymnastics and dance. Jim's wife works full time at a local agricultural plant. Jim is an active outdoors type who enjoys gardening, fishing, and bike riding. He is responsible for getting the kids off to school, taking care of the household, making dinner, and helping the kids with their homework when they return from school. Jim has experienced a major trauma in his life that will affect his role as a provider and have a negative impact on all of his occupational roles over the course of the next 12-16 weeks.

Jim was referred to occupational therapy by his orthopedic surgeon following an accident at work. Jim does not know exactly what caused the accident, but when he reached over to remove a small part wedged in the press, the press fired. The press came down squarely on the dorsal surface of his dominant right hand, crushing the dorsal aspect of the hand and lacerating the extensor tendons of his index, middle, and ring fingers.

Jim is still shaken when he talks about the accident and the subsequent surgery to repair his tendons. The physician immobilized the digits for almost 2 weeks secondary to a wound infection, and unfortunately Jim waited an additional week to schedule an occupational therapy appointment. Jim's hand is discolored, edematous, and painful, with limited functional or passive movement. Although he is thankful that he did not lose his fingers, Jim's life and roles have dramatically changed. Jim wants to know if he will ever be able to use his hand again or return to work. The Workers' Compensation coordinator as well as the orthopedic surgeon ask the same question.

How do we facilitate healing to expedite the return to occupational roles in so traumatic an injury? One approach is to incorporate therapeutic ultrasound into the traditional treatment. Jim's case is not unusual for many occupational therapists treating orthopedic injuries. The approach that we as occupational therapists use with these types of patients is unique, however. It is the occupational therapist's holistic focus and careful consideration of the media and methods used as part of the treatment process which places us in an excellent position to utilize physical technologies including therapeutic ultrasound as part of our treatment repertoire.

Jim's Response to Ultrasound

Jim presented with a number of deficit areas, including decreased tendon gliding over the metacarpophalangeal joints, wound infection with decreased healing, and an inability to perform functional activities and occupations requiring bilateral manipulation or lifting. Circumferential measurements, range of motion, grip and pinch strength, sensory testing, wound and scar evaluation, and assessment of functional activities were all component areas assessed and documented. His goals included increasing tendon gliding, increasing range of motion, improving prehension patterns and functional use of the hand, improving functional abilities, and returning to competitive employment and rates of production.

Therapeutic ultrasound was selected as an adjunct to Jim's treatment due to the small area of injury and because of the tendency for the collagen rich tendon and joint capsules to selectively "absorb" the sound energy. Because the tissue area was superficial, the ultrasound frequency selected was 3 MHz/0.2 W/cm, pulsed at 20% duty cycle for 5 minutes. The smallest transducer (2 cm) was selected to localize the sound energy. A low intensity was chosen because of the subacute nature of the condition and for the nonthermal benefits to facilitate the wound healing process. Low intensity was also used because of the reflection at the tissue-bone interface, which could increase the intensity by a small amount. Therapeutic ultrasound preceded active motion incorporating flexion and limited excursion, active and full passive movement into extension in order to enhance tendon gliding and to facilitate the healing process.

As Jim improved and as the treatment sessions progressed, measurement of change was documented, and ultrasound parameters were revised to achieve a thermal effect to facilitate tissue elongation. The frequency continued to be 3 MHz, but intensity was increased to 1.0 W/cm^2 at 100% duty cycle. The lifting requirements and prehension patterns needed to safely and effectively perform his job requirements also were incorporated into Jim's treatment plan.

Jim eventually returned to competitive employment, was able to play catch with his son again, and resumed his occupational roles as husband, father, provider, and caretaker of the children. Therapeutic ultrasound played an important and vital part of his overall treatment program.

Summary

Therapeutic ultrasound can be an effective adjunct in the occupational therapist's treatment repertoire. The ability of ultrasound to increase tissue extensibility, decrease pain and muscle spasm, and facilitate tissue healing and repair make it a vital addition to the treatment program for selected patients and conditions. The occupational therapist using ultrasound as an adjunct to treatment should have a thorough understanding of the physics, biophysical effects, precautions, and contraindications involved in order to achieve the maximum benefit of the effects of ultrasound.

References

1. Halliday D, Resnick R. *Physics*. New York: John Wiley & Sons; 1990.

2. Williams AR. *Ultrasound: Biological Effects and Potential Hazards*. London: Academic Press Inc. Ltd; 1983.

3. Buchtala V. The present state of ultrasonic therapy. *Br J Phys Med*. 1952;15:3.

4. Kuittert JH, Harr ET. Introduction to the clinical application of ultrasound. *Phys Ther Rev*. 1955;35:19.

5. Arnheim D. Therapeutic modalities. In: Arnheim D, ed. *Modern Principles of Athletic Training*. St. Louis, MO: Times Mirror/Mosby College Publishing; 1989:350-367.

6. Lehman J, Warren C, Guy A. *Ultrasound: Its Applications in Medicine and Biology*. New York: Elsevier Scientific; 1978.

7. Piersol GM, Schwann HP, Pennel RB, Carstensen EL. Mechanism of absorption of ultrasonic energy in blood. *Arch Phys Med Rehabil*. 1952;33:327-331.

8. Kimura I, Gulick D, Shelly J, Ziskin M. Effects of two ultrasound devices and angles of application on the temperature of tissue phantom. *JOSPT*. 1998;27:27-31.

9. Allen KGR, Battye CK. Performance of ultrasound therapy equipment in Pinellas county. *Phys Ther*. 1978;54:174-179.

10. Fyfe MC, Parnell SM. The importance of measurement of effective transducer radiating area in the testing and calibration of therapeutic ultrasonic instruments. *Health Phys*. 1982;43:377-381.

11. Hekkenberg RT, Oosterbaan WA, Van Beekum WT. Evaluation of ultrasound therapy devices. *Physiotherapy*. 1986;72(8):390-395.

12. Stewart HF, Abzug JL, Harris GH. Considerations in ultrasound therapy and equipment performance. *Phys Ther*. 1980;60(4):424-428.

13. Piersol GM, Schwan HP, Penwell RB, et al. Mechanism of absorption of ultrasonic energy in blood. *Arch Phys Med Rehabil*. 1952;33:327.

14. Wells PNT. Ultrasonics in medicine and biology. *Phys Med Biol*. 1977;22:629-669.

15. Binder A, Hodge G, Greenwood AM, Hazleman BL, Page Thomas DP. Is therapeutic ultrasound effective in treating soft tissue lesions. *Br Med J*. 1985;290:512-514.

16. Dyson M, Pond JB, Joseph J, Warwick R. The stimulation of tissue regeneration by means of ultrasound. *Clin Sci*. 1968;35:273-285.

17. Dyson M, Suckling J. Stimulation of tissue repair by ultrasound: a survey of mechanisms involved. *Physiotherapy*. 1978;64(4):105-108.

18. Enwemeka CS. The effects of therapeutic ultrasound on tendon healing. *Am J Phys Med Rehabil*. 1989;68(6):283-287.

19. Freider S, Weisberg J, Fleming B, Stanek A. A pilot study: The therapeutic effect of ultrasound following partial rupture of Achilles tendons in male rats. *J Orthop Sports Phys Ther*. 1988;10(2):39-45.

20. Dyson M, Pond JB. The effect of pulsed ultrasound on tissue regeneration. *Physiother*. 1970;64:105-108.

21. Apfel RE. Acoustic cavitation: A possible consequence of biomedical uses of ultrasound. *Br J Cancer*. 1989;45(suppl V):140.

22. Lehmann JF, Guy AW. Ultrasound therapy. In Reid J, Sikov MR, eds. *Interaction of Ultrasound and Biological Tissues*. Seattle, WA: DHEW Pub (FDA) 1971;73-8008: Session 3;8:141-152.

23. Lehmann JF, Herrick JF. Biologic reactions to cavitation, a consideration for ultrasonic therapy. *Arch Phys Med Rehabil*. 1953;34:86.

24. Dinno MA, Dyson M, Young SR, Mortimer AJ, Hart J, Crum LA. The significance of membrane changes in the safe and effective use of therapeutic and diagnostic ultrasound. *Phys Med Biol*. 1989;34(11):1543-1552.

25. Dyson, M. Role of ultrasound in wound healing. In: McCullough JM, Kloth LC, Feedar JA, eds. *Wound Healing: Alternatives in Management*. 2nd ed. Philadelphia, PA: FA Davis; 1995.

26. Heckman JD, Ryaby JP, McCabe J. Acceleration of tibial fracture healing by non-invasive, low intensity ultrasound. *J Bone Jt Surg*. 1994;76A(1) 26-34.

27. Pilla AA, Mont MA, Nasser PR. Non-invasive low intensity ultrasound accelerates bone healing in the rabbit. *J Orth Trauma*. 1990;4(3): 246-253.

28. Michlovitz S. *Thermal Agents in Rehabilitation*. 3rd ed. Philadelphia, Pa: F.A. Davis; 1996.

29. Reimann B. Ultrasound therapy: non-thermal effects on the inflammatory process. *Sports Medicine*. 1997:12;13-17.

30. Lehmann JF, et al. Effects of therapeutic temperatures on tissue extensibility. *Arch Phys Med Rehabil*. 1970;481:41.

31. Sapega AA, et al. Biophysical factors in range of motion excercise. *Physician Sports Med*. 1981;9:57.

32. Kramer JF. Ultrasound: Evaluation of its mechanical and thermal effects. *Arch Phys Med Rehabil*. 1984;65:223.

33. Draper DO. A comparison of temperature rise in human calf muscles following application of underwater and topical gel ultrasound. *J Orthop Phys Ther*. 1993;17:247.

34. Reid DC, Cummings GE. Factors in selecting the dosage of ultrasound with particular reference to the use of various coupling agents. *Phisiother Can*. 1973:63:255.

35. Wissiniger WI, Estervig DN, Wang RJ. A differential staining technique for simultaneous visualization of mitotic spindle and chromosomes in mamillian cells. *Stain Technology*. 1981;56:221-226.

36. De Deyne PG, Kirsch-Volders M. In vitro effects of therapeutic ultrasound on nucleum of human fibroblasts. *Phys Ther* 1995;75:629-633.

37. Sicard-Rosenbaum L, Lord D, Danoff JV, et al. Effects of continuous therapeutic ultrasound on growth and metastasis of subcutaneous murine tumors. *Phys Ther*. 1995;75:3-13.

38. Lehmann JF, et al. Ultrasound: considerations for use in the presence of prosthetic joints. *Arch Phys Med Rehabil*. 1980;61:502.

39. Skouba-Kristensen E. Ultrasound influence on internal fixation with a rigid plate in dogs. *Arch Phys Med Rehabil*. 1982;63:37.

40. Kotenber R, Ambrose L, Mosher R. Therapeutic ultrasound effect on high density polyethylene and polymethyl methacrylate. *Arch Phys Med Rehabil*. (abst) 1986;67:618.

41. Ter harr G. Recent advances and techniques in therapeutic ultrasound. In: Rapacholi MH, Grandolfo M, Rindi A, eds. *Ultrasound: Medical Applications, Biological Effects and Hazard Potential*. New York: Plenum Press;1987:333.

42. Masse J. Phonophoresis. *Sports Medicine*. 1996;10:4-6.

43. Franklin M, Smith S, Chenier T, Franklin R. Effect of phonophoresis with dexamethasone on adrenal function. *JOSPT*. 1995;22:103-107.

44. Byl N, McKenzie A, Halliday B, et al. The effects of phonophoresis with corticosteroids: a controlled pilot study. *JOSPT*. 1993;18:590-599.

45. Henley E. Transcutaneous drug delivery: iontophoresis, phonophoresis. *Critical Reviews in Physical Medicine and Rehabilitation*. 1991;3:139-151.

46. Byl NN. the use of ultrasound as an enhancer for transutaneous drug delivery: phonophoresis. *Phys Ther*. 1995:75:539-553.

47. Ciccone CD, Leggin BG, Callamaro JJ. Effects of ultrasound and trolamine salicylate phonophoresis. *Phys Ther*. 1991;71:666.

48. Cameron M, Monroe L. Relative transmission of ultrasound by media customarily used for phonorphoresis. *Phys Ther*. 1992;72:142-148.

Bibliography

Al-Karmi A. Calcium and the effects of ultrasound on frog skin. *Ultrasound Med Biol*. 1994;20:74.

Balmaseda MT. Ultrasound therapy: a comparative study of different coupling media. *Arch Phys Med Rehabil*. 1986;67:147.

Benson HAE, McElnay JC. Transmission of ultrasound through topic pharmaceutical products. *Physiotherapy*. 1988;74:587.

Benson HA, McElnay JC. Topical NSAID products as ultrasound couplants: their potential in phonophoresis. *Physiotherapy*. 1994;80:74.

Benson HA, McElnay JC, Harland R. Use of ultrasound to enhance percutaneous absorption of benzydamine. *Phys Ther*. 1989;69:114.

Brueton RN, Campbell B. The use of geliperm as a sterile coupling agent for therapeutic ultrasound. *Physiotherapy*. 1987;73:653.

Cook SD. Acceleration of tibia and distal radius fracture healing in patients who smoke. *Clinical Orthop*. 1997;337:198.

Docker MF, Foulkes DJ, Patrick MK. Ultrasound couplants for physiotherapy. *Physiotherapy*. 1982;68:124.

Holdsworth LK, Anderson DM. Effectiveness of ultrasound used with a hydrocortisone coupling medium or epicondylitis clasp to treat lateral epicondylitis: pilot study. *Physiotherapy*. 1993;79:19.

Klienkort JA, Wood F. Phonophoresis with 1% vs 10% hydrocortisone. *Phys Ther*. 1975;55:1321.

Lentell G, et al. The use of thermal agents to influence the effectiveness of a low-load prolonged stretch. *J Orthop Sports Phys Ther*. 1992;16:200.

Onate J. Ultrasound therapy: utilization in bone healing. *Sports Medicine*. 1997;12:18-21.

Sussman C, Dyson M. Therapeutic and diagnostic ultrasound. In: Sussman C, Bates B, eds. *Wound Care: A Collaborative Practice Manual for Physical Therapists and Nurses*. Aspen Publishers, Gaithersburg,Md: 1998.

Turner SM, Powell ES, Ng CSS. The effect of ultrasound on the healing of repaired cockeral tendon: is collagen cross linkage a factor? *J Hand Surgery*. 1989:14B(4):428-433.

Williams R. Production and transmission of ultrasound. *Physiotherapy*. 1987;73:113.

Young SR, Dyson M. The effect of therapeutic ultrasound on angiogenesis. *Ultrasound Med Biol*. 1990;16:261.

Chapter Seven
Trancutaneous Electrical Nerve Stimulation

Learning Objectives

1. Define TENS.
2. Describe the Gate Control Theory.
3. Discuss the Endorphin Theory.
4. Identify the types of stimulation programs available for use in TENS.
5. Outline clinical reasoning regarding the use of TENS with patient populations.

Terminology

Acupuncture Point
Conventional TENS
Electroacupuncture
Electrode
Endogenous Opiates
Gate Control Theory

Motor Point
Subsensory
Transcutaneous Electrical
    Nerve Stimulation
Trigger Point

TENS Theory

Transcutaneous electrical nerve stimulation (TENS) is the application of electrical stimulation for pain control. TENS is a generic term used to describe the process of applying controlled low voltage electrical pulses to the nervous system by passing electricity through electrodes which are placed on the skin. TENS was developed as a noninvasive technique of afferent stimulation to control pain.

There are a number of theories which have been postulated to explain how pain is transmitted. Many credit the work of Melzack and Wall for facilitating the development of TENS and pain theory with their Gate Control Theory in the mid 1960s. The two primary theories postulating the modulation of pain associated with TENS are the Gate Theory and the Endorphin Theory. Pain management involves controlling the perception and sensation of pain. Use of TENS as a component of pain management provides the therapist with a technology to provide an analgesic (absence of pain) effect, facilitating occupational performance.

Gate Theory

In the mid 1960s, Melzack and Wall described their Gate Theory of Pain, which stimulated the interest, development, and manufacture of TENS equipment, and facilitated further research into pain and pain perception. Melzack and Wall hypothesized that stimulation of nonnociceptors or their axons would interfere with the transmission of sensation from nociceptors to the higher centers of the brain where pain is perceived. Stimulation of the sensory A fibers with high-frequency TENS would flood the pathway to the brain and close the "gate" blocking the pain signal. As the body becomes habituated, more intense stimulation of the A fibers to keep the gate closed to the pain stimulus is required. The gate control system is thought to be located in a segment of the spinal cord known as the substantia gelatinosia in the specialized T-cells.[1-3]

Endorphin Theory

The second theory attributed to the effects of TENS is known as the Endorphin Theory. An extensive amount of research has come out of the field of neuropharmacology in the past 25 years, contributing greatly to understanding pain. Endorphin theory is based on the discovery of natural opiates which are pain suppressors in the body.[4,5] These endogenous opiates are the body's own natural pain relievers, and are produced by the pituitary gland and in the spinal cord. The pituitary gland produces beta-endorphins, and the spinal cord enkephalins. The neurohumeral/neurotransmitter theory suggests that TENS stimulates the body's production of these endogenous opiates which interact with receptors and block the perception of pain. These endogenous opiates are effective at decreasing the perception of pain, and mimic the action of narcotic drugs.[6-11]

Acupuncture Theory

An additional theory postulated to describe the effectiveness of TENS in the management of pain is related to the energy lines or meridians and acupuncture points associated with acupuncture. Some theorists believe that TENS can be used to stimulate the "entry" or acupuncture points along the same meridians used in traditional acupuncture with a resultant decrease in pain perception. Basic acupuncture points are highly innervated and vascularized regions of the body that may overlie the nerves at their superficial aspects. There are basic acupuncture points for a variety of pain syndromes which may lie on or adjacent to the site of pain or are distant from the site of pain. Acupuncture points are electrically active and exhibit a decreased resistance to the flow of electrical current. It is beyond the scope of this text to review the foundations of acupuncture and the interested reader is urged to research the topic further.[11-14]

Treatment Parameters of TENS

TENS has been used to manage pain in a variety of musculoskeletal disorders, including low back pain, arthritis, inflammatory disorders of soft tissue, postoperative pain, and other disease processes. There is some controversy and inconclusiveness with regard to the effectiveness of TENS, though inconsistencies in terminology and treatment parameters may account for the discrepancies. Treatment applications incorporating electrical stimulation for pain control employ pulsed or alternating currents with a variety of combinations of stimulation patterns. TENS equipment provides the clinician with a wide selection of parameters to choose. TENS technologies and equipment are generally characterized by the pulse amplitude, pulse duration or pulse width, and pulse frequency.[15,16]

There are four types of stimulation programs based on the neurological response to the stimulation either reported by the patient or observed in response to the stimulation. The four types of stimulation commonly used are subsensory level, sensory level, motor level, and noxious level.

Subsensory Level Stimulation

Subsensory level electrotherapy is also known commercially as MENS, or microcurrent electrical neuromuscular stimulation. Subsensory level TENS is also one of the most controversial TENS technologies. Subsensory level TENS assumes that microamperage (uA) currents are more effective at enhancing cellular physiology processes. The subsensory level stimulation produces currents consisting of the movement of ions in the biological tissues.[17-19] These currents are not of sufficient strength or magnitude, however, to produce a recognizable response in the nerve or muscle, and patients do not report any cutaneous sensation.

One of the underlying assumptions of subsensory stimulation is the belief that the body more comfortably and efficiently accepts this electrical energy into its own electrophysiological healing systems. Proponents also contend that the subsensory stimulation closely approximates the naturally occurring bioelectric current found in the body. The low-volt microamperage stimulation is within the range of the body's own physiological currents which enhances comfort and safety.[19-21] There is, however, little research evidence supporting the clinical efficacy of subsensory-level stimulation for pain or for wound healing, and the clinician should have some degree of skepticism toward manufacturers' claims.

Subsensory Level Parameters		
Pulse Duration:	**Frequency** (pps, bps, Hz):	**Amplitude:**
1 sec.	< 1mA	5-20 minute applications 1-3 x daily; subsensory, no noticeable motor or sensory response

Sensory Level Stimulation

Sensory level stimulation is also known as "conventional TENS", and consists of stimulation for pain control which is delivered at higher frequencies (50-100 pulse/sec). Conventional TENS is the most commonly used type of TENS and employs amplitudes and durations of stimulation which activate the cutaneous tactile sensory fibers. Stimulation produces a cutaneous paresthesia (pins and needles) or tingling sensation without muscle contraction, if the frequency of stimulation is greater than 10-15 pulses per second. Conventional TENS is based on the Gate Theory or counter irritation theory, and affects the large afferent (A) fibers, thereby influencing pain transmission.

If the frequency of stimulation is less than 7 to 10 pulses per second, patients experience a tapping sensation. The patient's sensory response increases if either the stimulus amplitude or pulse duration is increased. The most commonly held parameters for sensory level stimulation are in the higher frequencies (50-100 pulse/sec). Pulsed or alternating therapeutic currents stimulate the cutaneous sensory primary afferents without a motor response being elicited. Electrode placement should be on or near the location of reported pain. The patient should report a reduction or modulation of the pain response with the stimulation, but there is minimal residual analgesia with accommodation frequently occurring.[22] Because of this, manufacturers of these devices have developed units with current modulators to minimize accommodation during stimulation.

Sensory Level Parameters			
Pulse Duration:	**Frequency:**	**Treatment Time:**	**Amplitude:**
50-100 microsec.	80-100	15-30 minutes	Tingling, tapping, pins and needles

Conditions: Acute pain, pain associated with positional or dynamic stretch, joint mobilization techniques.

Motor Level Stimulation

Motor level stimulation occurs when the current becomes strong enough to activate the axons innervating skeletal muscle, causing muscle contractions. Motor level stimulation has also been termed strong low-rate (SLR) or acupuncture like TENS, based on the frequency of stimulation and the concurrent motor level stimulation. Dependent on the frequency stimulation, the tissue response can be one of tremo, or twitch-like contractions which occur when the frequency of stimulation is low (<5 pulse/sec), or the response can become smooth, isometric or isotonic tetanic contraction. Increasing the amplitude of the stimulation causes the muscle contractions to become stronger through recruitment of additional motor axons and/or muscle fibers.

Motor level stimulation is characterized by a high amplitude and low frequency, with a frequency below 10 pps, and typically in the range of 1-4 pps. Pulse duration is most often between a range from 100 to 300 usec (microseconds). The amplitude should be sufficient to produce strong, visible muscle contractions which may be uncomfortable to patients, but within their level of tolerance to discomfort. Pain reduction is thought to occur through the Gate Control Theory or due to endorphin release with the duration of analgesia lasting longer than other forms. Electrodes should be placed over the motor points which correlate with the location of pain or on the segmental nerve roots corresponding with the location of pain.[23-25]

Motor Level Parameters

Pulse Duration:	Frequency:	Treatment Time:	Amplitude:
150-200 microsec.	2-10	30-45 minutes	muscle twitch, tremor like, may be smooth, isometric or isotonic tetanic contraction

Conditions: Used for acute pain conditions and chronic pain conditions.

Noxious Level (Brief Intense) Stimulation

Noxious level stimulation is known by a number of pseudonyms, including electroacupuncture, hyperstimulation, or noxious level TENS. In all cases, when the stimulation amplitude is increased to a level which the patient perceives as painful, noxious level stimulation has been reached. Noxious stimulation is most often associated with the electrical activation of pain fibers near the site of stimulation. The parameters used for noxious level stimulation can produce a motor response, and areas containing superficial motor nerves or motor points should be avoided. Acupuncture meridians which correspond to the painful area can be used as the stimulation points. Brief intense (or noxious) stimulation uses high frequencies of 50-100 pulses/sec., with a pulse duration between 50-100 microseconds.

Noxious level stimulation is believed to modulate pain through the release of endogenous opiates. Noxious level stimulation produces a surface analgesia of short duration and can be used prior to passive stretch, debridement or minor surgery. Because noxious level stimulation produces an uncomfortable response, it should be used when other modes of TENS have been unsuccessful.

Noxious Level Parameters

Pulse Duration:	Frequency:	Treatment Time:	Amplitude:
1 ms-1 sec	1-5 or > 100	30 seconds per point	cutaneous paresthesia, noxious, may be painful

Conditions: Used for acute or chronic pain syndromes, before passive or positional stretching, burn debridement, or minor surgery.

Application and Efficacy

The literature is controversial and unclear on which method of TENS is more effective in the treatment of pain in patients. Use of TENS and the research that followed occured as an outgrowth of Wall and Melzack's Gate Theory. Early studies found that TENS use was promising for the reduction of low back pain and overall to modulate pain, but the research lacked consistent terminology and parameter selection, and had a variety of methodological and documentation errors and inconsistencies.[26,27]

Ordog[28] examined the analgesic effect of sensory level TENS on patients with acute traumatic conditions including sprains, lacerations, fractures, and contusions. He concluded that for acute injuries, active TENS alone was as effective as Tylenol with codeine in controlling posttraumatic pain. He suggested that active TENS might be the preferred method of pain control in order to avoid the sedative effects of narcotic anagesics. Paris[29] reported that monophasic-pulsed current stimulation of acupuncture points on patients with second degree ankle inversion sprains appeared to relieve pain faster than the standard treatment. Denegar and Huff[30] determined that high frequency TENS produced greater reduction in muscle induced soreness immediately after treatment than low frequency TENS. Denegar and Perrin[31] also found that TENS and cold produced significantly greater pain relief in delayed onset muscle soreness. Sensory and motor level forms of TENS have been shown to decrease muscle soreness pain which is often associated with acute inflammatory response. However, MENS, which is subsensory stimulation, does not appear to alter the magnitude of pain in acute inflammatory conditions such as lateral epicondylitis or elbow tendinitis.[32,33] There are no controlled studies demonstrating an analgesic effect of MENS for pain control in acute inflammatory conditions, and caution should be used when extrapolating manufacturers' claims for the equipment to clinical practice.[34,35] TENS has also been shown to be effective in the treatment of arthritis, tendinitis, adhesive capsulitis, and for the modulation of pain in aggressive active range of motion programs.[36-39]

Electrode Placement

Due to the variability regarding the most effective mode and parameters used for modulating pain in patients, therapists need to be flexible in their selection of TENS technologies and electrode locations. Stimulation sites for electrode placement should be selected based on the problem areas and goals selected for the patient. Optimal electrode placements should correlate with the initial evaluation which identified the structures and sources of pain. It is important for therapists to keep in mind the degree of skin resistance when selecting electrode sites. An area with greater resistance to the current may require a higher current which is uncomfortable for the patient. There are essentially three identifiable areas which are electrically active and can be used to facilitate current flow into the targeted tissue: motor points, trigger points, and acupuncture points.

Motor Points

Peripheral nerves which innervate a painful area and are located superficially can be targeted for direct stimulation. Motor points occur where the peripheral nerve enters the muscle and can also be used as a stimulation point. Less electrical current is necessary to cause a motor response at these areas. Motor points are located in the center of the muscle belly where the motor nerve enters the muscle and a visible contraction is elicited with a minimal amount of stimulation. If a muscle contraction or motor response is desired, electrodes should be placed over the motor point of the selected tissue. The frequency, pulse duration, and intensity should be adjusted to produce the desired clinical response, a muscle twitch, or a tetanic contraction.

Trigger Points

Areas which are hypersensitive to pressure and to electrical stimulation are known as trigger points, and can be located in the skin, fascia, muscle, tendon, ligament, or periosteum. Trigger points have a lower resistance to electrical activity and may be painful with compression. Palpation of the trigger point causes referred pain which radiates away from the area and does not always follow a segmental pattern. If the patient displays pain with palpation of the trigger point, the therapist can select the area for electrode placement. Electrodes can be placed over the trigger point or in relation to the zone of referred pain.

Acupuncture Points

Acupuncture points and the ancient Chinese meridians associated with them can also be used for pain management. Acupuncture points can be targeted along sequential, predefined points, or by treating successive points along the meridian that passes through the painful area. Acupuncture points are located over the entire body and there are a number of charts which have been mapped out to facilitate electrode placement. The acupuncture points and principles are based on thousands of years of Chinese tradition and are identified as meridians. These acupuncture points are highly innervated and vascularized areas which may overlie the nerves at their superficial locations. Electrodes can be placed on a single point or on multiple points concurrently. Stimulation using a predefined sequence of acupuncture points exhibiting a decreased pain threshold along the meridian that passes through the painful area can be also be used (Figure 7-1).

Electrodes

The most common adverse reaction to TENS or electrical stimulation is skin irritation. The irritation occurs at the skin-electrode interface and may occur with any of the wide variety of commercially available electrodes. Patients who have a sensitivity to adhesive products are the most susceptible. Incidents where patients demonstrate an allergic reaction to an adhesive polymer electrode or who are sensitive and react to the metal snap projection in the center of an electrode should be reported to the manufacturer of the electrodes.

There are a variety of electrode types and sizes that are available, and there is not just one type of electrode that is right for every patient. The primary types of electrodes available include carbon rubber, gel type, or self-adhering. The carbon rubber and gel types of electrodes require the clinician to use a conductive gel and to tape the electrode to the targeted area. Self-adhering electrodes may be single-use or reusable.

Figure 7-1. Auriculo-therapy points (acupuncture). Illustration by Kim Bartlett. Used with permission.

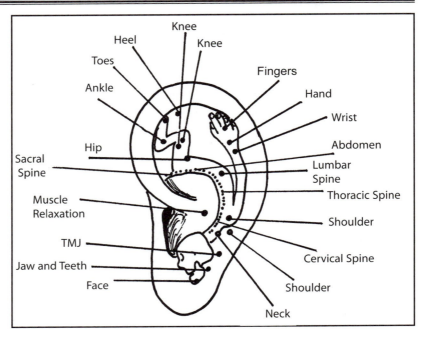

Patient compliance is usually better when these types of electrodes are used. As a general rule, larger electrodes are used for generalized pain or for multiple electrode set-ups. Smaller electrodes are best used for deep localized pain, and smaller self-adhering electrodes may adhere better in certain areas of the body. The density of the current is determined by the size of the electrode, with a smaller electrode possessing greater density and producing a greater sensation.

It is vital that the skin is cleaned prior to application of the electrodes. The skin should be washed with water and soap, rinsed, and then blotted dry. Large electrodes should be used on the larger areas of the body such as the back or leg, and smaller sizes used on smaller areas, such as the face and hand. The therapist should use different size electrodes where muscle contractions are easily elicited or hypersensitivity occurs.

Skin burns may occur with excessive stimulation to an area. Burns are more likely to occur with the use of small-area electrodes and care should be used to avoid placing any size electrode too close to another. If there is poor electrical contact between the skin and the electrode, micropunctate burns may occur. Skin irritation and burns may be caused by an improperly applied electrode which does not conform to the contour of the area, or the electrode may lack gel or be too dry. Mechanical stresses caused by the shearing forces between the tape and the skin when the electrodes are removed may also cause an adverse skin reaction. Care should be used when applying tape, and the electrodes should be removed from the skin with the movement occurring in the direction that the hair in the region lies. Skin integrity is crucial for effective transmission of the electrical current and should be clean and clear of lesions. Therapists should always carefully inspect the skin for any cuts or disruptions of skin integrity and ensure that the area has normal sensation.

Electrode Placement

There appears to be a relationship between motor, trigger, and acupuncture points. All are resistant to palpation and can be painful or tender with referred pain. All of these points are electrically active and exhibit a decreased resistance to the flow of electrical energy. This decreased impedance facilitates the flow of electrical current into the tissue and the body. The therapist must be able to identify whether the desired outcome involves a motor response, sensory analgesia, or noxious stimulation for analgesia. For initial placement, electrodes can be placed over or contiguous to the site of pain. Stimulation sites also include the tissue overlying the painful area, the superficial points along the peripheral nerves, the specific dermatomes or spinal segmental myotomes, trigger points, motor points, or acupuncture points. The therapist should monitor the patient's response to the stimulation and move the electrodes to a different site if desired results do not occur.

There are a variety of electrode placements and patterns which can be used with TENS. There are no hard and fast rules regarding electrode arrangements, and therapists should be willing to change their initial electrode placements if the treatment outcomes are less than expected or if the patient experiences pain or discomfort. Electrodes can be placed parallel to the painful site or on either side of a scar or surgical incision; crossed at the site of localized pain; bracketed, which places the electrodes outside the margins of the painful area; or linear, which places the electrodes along the distribution of referred pain, along a peripheral nerve or dermatome. Electrode patterns can be unilateral, bilateral, or contralateral. Electrode patterns which have all electrodes located on the same side of the joint, spine, face, or extremity are referred to as unilateral. Bilateral electrode placements occur when the electrodes are placed on both sides of a peripheral joint, spine, face, or if the opposite extremity sites are used. Contralateral electrode placement is best used when the painful area is irritable or hyperesthetic and inaccessible (see Appendix).

Contraindications

Though TENS and electrical stimulation devices provide a safe and effective technology, care should be taken when using electrical stimulation for pain management with some patients, and it is contraindicated for some specific diagnoses and areas (Table 7-1).

TENS units should not be used with demand type cardiac pacemakers as it may interfere with their function and performance. Though electroanalgesia has been used during labor and delivery, the FDA recommends that it not be performed on the trunk or abdomen of pregnant women. Electroanalgesia should also not be applied directly over the eye, in individuals with epilepsy or malignancies, with patients with peripheral vascular disease or infection, or those with a loss of or decreased sensation. Electroanalgesia has been used for pain control with patients who have been diagnosed with terminal cancer, but informed consent of the patient should be obtained prior to treatment implementation. TENS is also contraindicated in patients with undiagnosed pain, and electrodes should not be placed over the carotid sinus area or transcerebrally. Caution should be used when using electroanalgesia on patients with acute pain or immediately postoperatively because the pain serves as a protective function to prevent or to warn of further damage to the tissue or body. TENS use may suppress the sensation of pain which functions as a protective mechanism. As with any medical device or medication, TENS devices should be kept out of the reach of children.

Table 7-1.
Contraindications

- demand-type pacemakers
- placement over carotid sinus
- pregnant patients during first trimester
- anterior neck area
- cardiac disease (stimulation across the chest)
- epilepsy (avoid head & neck area)
- placement over the eyes
- mucosal surfaces
- patients with central nervous system disorders
- patients with CVAs
- confused or noncompliant patients
- children

Clinical Reasoning and Application

As with any technology, TENS is used as a part of the overall treatment process. TENS can be a safe and effective adjunct or alternative to traditional pharmacological or surgical interventions when used to modulate pain and facilitate occupational performance. TENS is, however, only one component of the pain modulation continuum. There is a wide variety of equipment, electrode placements, and parameters available, and therapists must be flexible and creative in selecting and applying the technology. As with any intervention, patient compliance and understanding of the treatment and the role TENS may play as a response to the injury or healing process is vital if effective outcomes are to occur.

A thorough evaluation should be completed before the application of TENS to ensure that the intervention is appropriate and indicated for the existing condition. A review of the patient's medical history, pain medications, and a thorough assessment of the patient's presenting condition, including the stage of recovery and level and area of pain, assists in determining treatment alternatives and parameters. The type of pain, length of healing, and psychological reaction and behavior to pain are important characteristics for consideration in the reasoning process. If a patient complains of chronic, generalized pain which is poorly localized and is in response to an injury which occurred months or years ago, the likelihood of positive outcomes for pain modulation using TENS is unlikely.

Obtaining a thorough understanding of the individual's occupational performance and the components involved is vital to assist in pain modulation and for preparation for resumption of occupational activities. There are a variety of pain scales available, such as the McGill Pain Questionnaire, and consistent administration of the pain scale assists in determining changes in pain. Before incorporating TENS as part of the treatment protocol, it is important to explain to the patient that TENS itself cannot cure the underlying problem, nor is it the magic answer to their pain. Patients who adopt a positive attitude toward the technology and assume responsibility for the intervention will facilitate more positive outcomes.

TENS stimulation is composed of different variables, including pulse rate, pulse width, and intensity. There is no universal agreement as to the optimal TENS mode or electrode placement for a given diagnosis or pathology. Patients, however, do appear to prefer and tolerate low-amplitude conventional TENS, and lower-amplitude formats of other modes such as brief intense, pulse-burst, or modulated.

As there are no hard and fast rules governing selection of a specific TENS format, using conventional mode TENS or presetting the duration low and the frequency high are appropriate starting points.[40-42] Electrodes should be bracketed around the area of pain, or proximal to or on the localized area of pain. When the unit is turned on, the amplitude should be increased until the patient reports a tingling sensation. If there is a good working relationship with the patient and he is accepting of the technology, the patient can adjust the amplitude, self-modulating the sensation and amplitude to the desired sensation. The patient should report a tingling sensation with paresthesia. No muscle response should be noted. Before turning on the TENS, the therapist should pre-set the pulse duration and frequency. Frequency should be set between 50-80 pps, with pulse duration between 50-100 milliseconds. Treatment duration should be a minimum of 20 minutes and a maximum of 60 minutes. Patients should be monitored throughout the course of the treatment with minor adjustments of the stimulation characteristics made as needed.

As with any technology, treatment should be discontinued immediately if the patient is in any distress, or if the patient is unable to tolerate the input. If the patient is able to tolerate the sensation and reports a decrease in pain with an improvement in functional movements, continuation of the stimulation is warranted. If the patient is unable to tolerate the stimulation or is not receiving any decrease in pain, changing the location of the electrodes or readjusting the stimulation parameters may improve the outcome. If the patient continues to complain of discomfort, a different form of TENS should be considered. Other modes of TENS stimulation include acupuncture-like (strong low rate) TENS, brief intense TENS, burst mode (pulse trains) TENS, or hyperstimulation (point stimulation) TENS.

Acupuncture-like or strong low rate TENS can be used to provide pain modulation during a chronic phase of pain. Amplitude setting should be strong, yet with a comfortable rhythmic muscle twitch. Frequency is between 1-5 pps with a pulse duration of 150-300 milliseconds. Treatment duration is between 30-40 minutes.

Brief intense TENS may be used for short-term pain relief and may be most effective prior to painful procedures such as joint mobilization, passive stretch, friction massage, or wound debridement. The amplitude is set to the patient's tolerance, with a frequency between 80-150 pps, and a pulse duration between 50-250 milliseconds. Treatment duration is usually short, up to 15 minutes.

The burst mode, or pulse trains TENS, provides characteristics of both high and low rate TENS and may be more tolerable to some patients. The amplitude is set to provide a tingling or paresthesia, with a frequency between 50-100 pps, which is cycled in bursts of 1-4 pps. The pulse duration is between 50-200 milliseconds and the length of the treatment is between 20-30 minutes. Pain relief is usually long lasting with this type of stimulation.

Point stimulation or hyperstimulation TENS is used to locate and to stimulate acupuncture or trigger points to a noxious level. As trigger points or acupuncture sites are being targeted, multiple sites may be stimulated depending upon the technique used. The amplitude is strong, and set to the patient's tolerance. Frequency varies from

1-5 pps with the pulse duration between 150-300 milliseconds. The stimulation continues for 15-30 seconds at each point.

Following the treatment, patients should be reevaluated to determine any significant change in their pain level and occupational performance. Use of a pain scale or pain log can assist the patient in tracking changes and assist in determining how long the pain modulation is lasting. Treating acute pain is generally more effective than treating chronic pain and quicker results are seen. Most often, patients will need to use the TENS units at home and they should be receptive and responsible to the use of the equipment. Verbal and written home program instructions should be provided to the patient. Having the patient demonstrate correct use of the equipment in the clinic is necessary. All parameters and controls should be demonstrated to the patient and to any other significant others or family members in order to facilitate patient compliance. Electrode preparation and placement should be reviewed, and anatomical placements can be highlighted in marker for the patient. Precautions and contraindications should be reviewed and summarized with the patient as well as being documented. A mechanism should be established for patient contact with the department/therapist in case difficulties are encountered, and as with any technology, formative evaluation and specific reevaluation dates should be established prior to the equipment being sent home with the patient.

Documentation

Documentation for TENS use should include the treatment parameters being utilized, electrode placements, and documentation of any pain scales and drawings. Changes in the patient's condition and subjective reports of sensation during and after the stimulation should be recorded, as well as the type of electrical stimulation, mode of delivery, pulse duration, frequency, intensity, and duration of treatment. Use of a descriptive pain scale or numerical rating scale on a consistent basis aids in reevaluation and adjustments in treatment parameters. Identifying any objective changes in occupational performance and occupational components such as range of motion, improved tolerance or engagement in an activity assist in determining efficacy of the intervention and patient compliance.

Summary

TENS can be an important adjunct to treatment interventions with patients experiencing pain. Pain is a multifaceted symptom which requires creativity and skill on the part of the therapist to decrease it and facilitate occupational functioning. Because of the variety of equipment, electrode placements, and approaches available to the therapist, patience and persistence in utilizing different TENS modes may be necessary to obtain optimal outcomes for the patient. Careful evaluation and monitoring of the patient's condition is necessary to determine modulation in pain and improvement in occupational performance.

Case Study

Mrs. M is an active 67 y/o female who was referred for occupational therapy with a diagnosis of status post (s/p) right Colles' fracture, her dominant hand. The injury occurred as a result of a fall from the bottom stair with the patient landing on her flexed wrist. Mrs. M has had the right extremity immobilized in a cast for 6 weeks. The cast was removed 5 days ago.

The patient's primary complaints since removal of the cast are "stiffness" and "pain at level 6" on a 1-10 pain scale. She has had difficulty "doing anything for myself, even holding onto the fork with my right hand", and the injury and subsequent pain and stiffness have limited her ability to perform basic activities of daily living requiring bilateral movement or stabilization, or any dominant hand activities requiring lifting or prehension. She also complains of her elbow and shoulder "aching" and feeling "stiff and sore". Sensation is intact, though she keeps the extremity in a flexed and guarded position. After evaluating the patient for active movement, AROM and PROM measurements, and circumferential measurements, noting any trophic changes or variations in skin temperature, and examining her x-rays, she is placed on an active treatment program. Assessment reveals that the impaired function and limitation in occupational performance is due to the fracture and immobilization of the wrist, resulting in pain, swelling, stiffness, and limited motion. Treatment plan includes whirlpool in the initial phase of therapy, ultrasound, gentle joint mobilization, engagement in occupational tasks requiring bilateral hand use and prehension patterns for the right, and slow, gentle passive stretching.

Because the patient reports pain following therapeutic interventions that are stressing the tissue at the end range of motion, and after functional activities, TENS is used as a posttreatment modality with the goal being to decrease the pain. This technology can also be incorporated into the home program to decrease pain, thereby facilitating occupational performance.

References

1. Melzack R, Wall PD. Pain mechanisms: a new theory. *Science*. 1965;150:971-977.

2. Melzack R,Wall PD. The gate control theory of pain. In: Soulairac A, Cahn J, Carpentier J, eds. *Pain: Proceedings of the International Symposium on Pain*. London: Academic Press; 1968.

3. Jessel TM, Kelly DD. Pain and analgesia. In: Kandel ER, Schwartz JH, Jessel TM eds. *Principles of Neural Science*. 3rd ed. New York: Elsevier; 1991:385-399.

4. Bonica JJ. *The Management of Pain, Vols I and II*. 2nd ed. Malvern, PA: Lea & Febiger; 1990.

5. Kandel ER, Schwartz JH, Jessell TM. *Principles of Neural Science* 3rd ed. New York: Elsevier; 1991.

6. Hughes J. Search for the endogenous legend of the opiate receptor. *Neurosci Res Program Bull.* 1975;13:55.

7. Hughes J. Intrinsic factors and the opiate receptor system. *Neurosci Res Program Bull.* 1978; 16:141

8. Salar G, Job I, Mingrino S. Effect of transcutaneous electrotherapy on CSF betaendorphin content in patients without pain problems. *Pain*. 1984; 10:169-172.

9. Basbaum A, Fields HL. Endogenous pain control systems: Brainstem spinal pathways and endorphin circuitry. *Annual Rev Neurosci*. 1984;7:309.

10. Duggan AW. The differential sensitivity to L-glutamate and L-asparate of spinal interneuronsand Renshaw cells. *Exp Brain Res*. 1974;19:522.

11. Elde R. Immunohistochemical studies using antibodies to leucine-enkephalin: Initial observations on the nervous system of the rat. *Neuroscience*. 1976;1:349.

12. Headley B. EMG and myofascial pain. *Clin Manag*. 1990;10:43.

13. Mann F. Acupuncture: *The Chinese Art of Healing and How it Works Scientifically*. New York: Vintage Books; 1973.

14. Melzack R, Stillwell D, Fox E. Trigger points and acupuncture points for pain: correlations and implications. *Pain*. 1977;3: 3-23.

15. Robinson AJ, Snyder-Mackler L, eds. *Clinical Electrophysiology: Electrotherapy and Electrophysiologic Testing*. 2nd ed. Baltimore, MD: Williams & Wilkins; 1995.

16. Low J, Reed A. Electrotherapy Explained: *Principles and Practice* 2nd ed. London: Butterworth-Heinemann; 1995.

17. Lerner F, Kirsch D. A double-blind comparative study of micro-stimulation and placebo effect: In short-term treatment of the chronic back pain patient. *ACA Journal of Chiropractic*. 1981;15:101-106.

18. Cheng N. The effects of electrical currents of ATP generation, protein synthesis, and membrane transport in rat skin. *Clinical Orthopedics*. 1982;11: 264-272.

19. Carley P, Wainapel S. Electrotherapy for acceleration of wound healing: low intensity direct current. *Archives of Phys Med and Rehab*. 1985;66:443-445.

20. Morgareidge K, Chipman R. Microcurrent therapy. *Physical Therapy Today*. 90;2:50-53.

21. Davis P. Microcurrent: A modern healthcare modality. *Rehab and Therapy Products Review*. 1992;11:62-66.

22. Rossen J. Managing pain with microcurrent stimulation. *PT Today*. 1995;3/13:4-7.

23. Mannheimer JS, Lampe GN. *Clinical transcutaneous electrical nerve stimulation*. Philadelphia, PA: F.A. Davis; 1984.

24. Manneheimer C, Lund S, Carlsson C. The effect of transcutaneous electrical nerve stimulation (TENS) on joint pain in patients with rheumatoid arthritis. *Scand J Rheumatol*. 1978;7:13-16.

25. Langley GB, Sheppeard H, Johnson M, Wigley RD. The analgesic effects of transcutaneous electrical nerve stimulation and placebo in chronic pain patients. A double-blind noncrossover comparison. *Rheumatol Int*. 1984;4:119-123.

26. Zizic TM, Hoffman KC, Holt PA, Hugerford DS, et al. The treatment of osteoarthritis of the knee with pulsed electrical stimulation. *J Rheumatol*. 1995;22: 1757-1761.

27. Robinson, AJ. Transcutaneous electrical nerve stimulation for the control of pain in musculoskeletal disorders. *Journal of Orthop & Sports Phys Ther*. 1996;24:208-226.

28. Ordog GJ. Transcutaneous electrical nerve stimulation versus oral analgesic: A randomized double blind controlled study in acute traumatic pain. *Am J Emerg Med*. 1987;5:6-10.

29. Paris DL, Baynes F, Gucker B. Effects of neuroprobe in the treatment of second degree ankle inversion sprains. *Phys Ther*. 1983;83(1):35-40.

30. Denegar CR, Huff CB. High and low frequency TENS in treatment of induced musculoskeletal pain: A comparison study. *Athl Train*. 1988;23:235-237, 258.

31. Denegar CR, Perrin DH. Influence of transcutaneous electrical nerve stimulation, cold, and a combination treatment on pain, decreased range of motion, and strength loss associated with delayed onset muscle soreness. *J Athl Train*. 1992;27:200-206.

32. Johannsen F, Gam A, et al. Rebox: An adjunct in physical medicine? *Arch Phys Med Rehabil*. 1993;74:438-440.

33. Robinson A. Transcutaneous electrical nerve stimulation for the control of pain in musculoskeletal disorders. *JOSPT*. 1996;24:208-226.

34. Fedorczyk J. The role of physical agents in modulating pain. *J Hand Ther*. 1997;10:110-121.

35. Mannheimer C, Lund S, Carlsson CA. The effect of transcutaneous electrical nerve stimulaiton in patients with rheumatoid arthritis: a comparative study of different pulse patterns. *Scand J Rheumatol*. 1978;7:13.

36. Mannheimer C, Carlsson CA. The analgesic effect of transcutaneous electrical nerve stimulation in patients with rheumatoid arthritis: a comparative study of different pulse patterns. *Pain*.

1979;6:329.

37. Rizk TE, Christopher RP, et al. Adhesive capsulitis (frozen shoulder): a new approach to its management. *Arch Phys Med.* 1983;64:29-33.

38. Cannon NM. Enhancing flexor tendon glide through tenolysis and hand therapy. *J Hand Ther.* 1989;3:122-137.

39. Andersson SA. Pain control by sensory stimulation. In: Bonica JJ, Liebeskind JC, Albe Fessard DG, eds. *Advances in Pain Research and Therapy.* New York: Raven Press; 1979:3;569-585.

40. Leo K. Perceived comfort levels of modulated versus conventional TENS current. *Phys Ther.* 1984;64:745.(abstract)

41. Barr JO, Weissenbuehler SA, Bandstra EJ, et al. Effectiveness and comfort level of transcutaneous electrical nerve stimulation (TENS) in elderly with chronic pain. *Phys Ther.* 1987;67:775. (abstract)

42. Paxton SL. Clinical uses of TENS: A survey of physical therapists. *Phys Ther.* 1980;60:38.

43. Barr JO, Nielsen DH, Soderberg GL. Transcutaneous electrical nerve stimulation characteristics for altering pain perception. *Phys Ther.* 1986;66:1515.

44. Linzer M, Long DM. Transcutaneous neural stimulation for relief of pain. *IEEE Trans Biomed Eng.* 1976;23:341.

Chapter Eight

Iontophoresis

Learning Objectives

1. Describe the clinical applications for iontophoresis.
2. Discuss the physical concepts and mechanisms related to the transdermal delivery of medication.
3. Describe the physical concepts and terminology of ion movement.
4. Identify common medications used in iontophoresis treatment.
5. Outline clinical decision-making regarding the indications and precautions in the use of iontophoresis as part of the treatment process.

Terminology

Anode	Ion Transfer
Cathode	Iontophoresis
Dermis	Polarity
Dosage	Stratum Corneum
Epidermis	Transdermal

Iontophoresis is a method of topically delivering medication or ionized drugs into a localized area of tissue by using the force of direct electrical current to create a therapeutic effect. Iontophoresis is a safe and effective way to administer medication because it is painless, sterile, and relatively noninvasive. Iontophoresis is used by a number of health care professionals in dentistry, dermatology, otorhinolaryngology, and ophthalmology to treat a variety of conditions.[1,2]

Occupational therapists frequently utilize iontophoresis to treat inflammatory conditions. It is important for the occupational therapist to have a basic understanding of the mechanism underlying iontophoresis to safely and effectively use it as an adjunct to treatment. Additionally, the occupational therapist should possess a fundamental grounding in the wound healing process and the pathophysiology of the specific diagnoses which are to be treated with iontophoresis. The occupational therapist must also be cognizant of the wide variety of medications and their therapeutic and physiological effects as well as the method of application to ensure a positive clinical outcome.

History

Iontophoresis is the process of introducing a topically applied medication into the epidermis or mucous membranes of selected tissue.[3] Literature related to iontophoresis dates as far back as the late 1700s and 1800s. The concept of iontophoresis and ion transfer has been in existence and in use since LeDuc discovered in 1908 that ions could be driven across the skin through the application of an electrical current.[4] Iontophoresis has grown in popularity with the advent of technological advances of miniaturization and computerization of equipment, as well as the development of effective electrodes to contain the chemicals.

In the past, difficulty with electrodes, lack of electrical safety, and lack of standardization of equipment causing an increased risk of burns, and inhibited the widespread use of iontophoresis in the clinic. With greater research and a better understanding of the mechanisms involved in iontophoresis, the risk to the patient has decreased and application of the treatment technique have grown. Uses for iontophoresis include administration of local anesthesia, topical application of antibiotics, and most commonly for occupational therapists, administration of drugs and steroids.

Biophysiology

Transdermal drug delivery has been widely used in the past to introduce various medications into selected tissue through the skin which is the outer layer of the body. Because of certain characteristics of the skin and its permeability, not all medications can be effectively administered this way. The skin effectively acts as a barrier, allowing very few drugs or chemicals to be delivered through the skin. To overcome this barrier and facilitate the movement of the drugs into the tissue, iontophoresis is used.

Skin is approximately 3 to 5 mm thick and is composed of three layers: the epidermis, dermis, and hypodermis. The primary impediment to the effective penetration of the drug through the skin is the stratum corneum. The stratum corneum is the lipid-rich outer most layer of the epidermis.[5] If the medication is able to penetrate this layer, it then becomes able to passively diffuse into the underlying subcutaneous tissue. There are two primary methods that allow the drug access to the underlying tissue: movement between the intercellular matrix, and through the normal openings of the skin.

The skin is relatively permeable to lipophilic or lipid soluble chemicals and acts as a barrier to water-soluble or hydrophilic substances. This lipid layer can be envisioned as the "mortar" between bricks. Small lipophilic molecules are able to pass through this intercellular matrix. The openings found in the normal openings of the skin, such as through the hair follicles, sweat, and sebaceous glands provide a second entrance into the body for chemicals. Hair follicles, sweat glands, and sebaceous glands extend deeper through the epidermis, into the dermis, and are more permeable and proximal to the vascular supply. Applying direct current to the skin assists in moving the chemicals into the subcutaneous tissue. [6]

Basic Principles

The outer layer of the epidermis, the stratum corneum, is composed of cells called *corneocytes*, which are separated by free fatty acids creating a lipid environment. Because of this composition, the stratum corneum becomes an effective barrier to water and other ionic substances, effectively keeping water within the body and preventing foreign material from entering. Iontophoresis delivers ionic drugs across this barrier because the charged drugs help to carry the current to complete an electrical circuit. Essentially, the direct electrical current moves the ions in a particular direction. The primary physics principle that makes iontophoresis successful is that like charges repel and opposite charges attract. The charged drugs are repulsed by an electrode of the same charge. This can be visualized if you recall taking two magnets and placing the same end together, positive:positive, negative:negative. When the magnets are placed same end-to-end, the ends of the magnet push the like charged end of the magnet away.

Ions possessing a positive charge can be moved into the epidermis by the positive electrode, and ions which possess a negative charge are propelled by the negative electrode. The negatively charged electrode is known as the cathode, repelling negatively charged ions. The positively charged electrode is known as the anode, repelling positively charged ions. When the electrical current is applied to the electrodes and medication, it repels the negative or positive ions away from the common pole toward the opposite pole facilitating the movement of the ions into the underlying tissue.[7,8] When the medication molecules have crossed the outer layer of the skin, the stratum corneum, the drug proceeds to disperse to all local tissues with the highest concentration of the medication being located in the tissues closest to the treatment (electrode) site. Concentrations of the medication are decreased the further away from the electrode.

The effectiveness of iontophoresis is dependent on the number of ions transferred, the depth of penetration, the combining of ions chemically with other substances in the skin, and the ability of the individual ion to enter the body.[9,10] Ion penetration extends approximately 1 mm below the electrode surface. The chemical effects from the introduced medication will extend to deeper levels by capillary action and through the biophysical conductance of the current.[11]

Application

The typical iontophoresis unit consists of a power source, a "working" or medicated electrode, and an indifferent electrode. Commercially available units such as Empi's

Dupel (Empi, Inc., St. Paul, Mn) and Iomed's Phoresor (Iomed, Inc., Salt Lake City, UT) are small battery powered units which deliver a direct current adjustable by the therapist. The working electrode consists of a chamber where the drug is contained. The indifferent electrode completes the circuit of current. The polarity of the active or medicated electrode should consist of the same polarity of the medication desired to deliver to the tissue. Though there is some passive diffusion of the oppositely charged ions, it is not as effective as using the appropriate pole. Like poles repel, and unlike poles attract.

The size of the ion also influences the ion delivery. Smaller ions with a lighter molecular weight have a tendency to move quicker and more freely. Larger ions move slower and may be too large to be effectively used with iontophoresis.[12,13] The anode (+) produces an acid reaction, with the cathode (-) producing an alkaline reaction. The anode, which is positive, is sclerotic, which hardens tissue and acts as an analgesic. The negatively charged cathode is sclerolytic, which is a softening agent and can be used clinically for the management of scars and burns. Most of the commercial electrode pads, such as Empi Corporation, use buffered pads which decrease the acid/alkali buildup at the anode and cathode and could cause chemical burns due to excessive buildup of the chemicals.

Dosage

In iontophoresis, dosage is measured in milliamp-minutes, the milliamps of the current multiplied by the minutes, or length of treatment. Dosage = Milliamps x Mins. There are two primary variables affecting the number of ions transported to the tissue, the current amplitude (dosage = mA x mins), and the duration of the current flow (dosage = mA x min). It is not the volume of the fluid or medication which is being delivered to the underlying tissue, but the ions which are being transported. The volume of the medication being measured into the electrode reservoir does not directly affect the number of ions which are transported, nor does the size of the electrode. Increasing the size of the medicated electrode effectively increases the total treatment area, however, the amount of medication delivered will be the same. The amount of drug delivered to the tissue is determined by the current and the duration of the treatment (current x time). The volume of medication, assuming it is of the same concentration, will not affect the amount of ions delivered. The significant variables affecting dosage are the current and duration.

It is not the total current, but the current density, which determines if a small, safe, and comfortable amount of current is being applied.[14] Most of the commercial units available deliver a maximum current of 4 mA. Therapists should use caution in ramping up the maximum current to avoid the possibility of the patient having an allergic reaction to the direct current, known as a galvanic rash. Galvanic rash may occur in those patients with a hypersensitivity to direct current. Ramping up the current too quickly may also be uncomfortable to the patient.

Current density is dependent on the surface area of the electrode and is determined by dividing the current amplitude by the total area of the electrode. To prevent skin irritation or burning, a lower current density such as $0.5 \ mA/cm^2$, should be used and is effective in transmitting the medication. Many protocols use a current density from 2 mA up to 4 mA, and the clinician should set the parameters based on client tolerance and comfort rather than speed of treatment. There has been some question whether the medication is able to cross the skin barrier and reach a therapeutic level when driven into the tissue quicker than 15 minutes.[15] Further research is necessary to determine the most effective treatment times. A good rule of thumb is to set the current density to patient tolerance, most often making the treatment time between 20-30 minutes. There are a number of manufacturers making electrodes and iontophoresis units including: Iomed's Phoresor, Empi's Dupel, Life-Tech's Iontophor, (Lifetech, Inc., Stafford, Tx) and Henley International's Dynaphor (Henley Intl., Sugarland, Tx).

Indications

Iontophoresis is an effective method of intervention which can be applied to a variety of conditions typically treated by occupational therapists. Most often, iontophoresis is used in the treatment of inflammatory conditions. Equipment manufacturers and researchers have identified a number of other diagnoses and interventions for which iontophoresis is effective including local anesthesia to decrease joint pain and inflammation, and for musculoskeletal inflammatory conditions.[16-18] Conditions most frequently seen by occupational therapists and which respond well to the medications and intervention include: carpal tunnel syndrome, epicondylitis, ulnar nerve inflammation, elbow strain/sprain, radio-humeral bursitis, triceps tendinitis, gleno-humeral bursitis, hand and wrist tendinitis/tenosynovitis, and DeQuervain's disease. Some manufacturers have developed diagnosis specific treatment and medication protocols which may be utilized in patient care, however, treatment parameters should always be specific to the patient and the therapist should understand the underlying patho-physiology of the disease and the medications used. It should also be noted that many of the protocols and reports lack the control of structured research, are anecdotal and should be used with caution.

Medications

Dexamethasone iontophoresis is perhaps the most widely applied medication used by therapists due to its antiinflammatory action. Iontophoresis has been shown to relieve pain and inflammation in tendinitis, osteoarthritis, synovitis, and patellofemoral joint and musculoskeletal problems, and in reducing scar tissue.[19-23] Use of local anesthetics such as lidocaine for pain relief is also a common technique used by the therapist and is based, in part, on anecdotal evidence and research in dentistry and otolaryngology (ears, nose, throat). Combining the antiinflammatory benefits of dexamethasone with the anesthetic function of lidocaine is frequently employed. There is, however, some controversy as to the effectiveness of this combination due to the negative polarity of the dexamethasone and the positive polarity of the lidocaine.[24-26] With co-iontophoresis of medications, switching the polarity during the treatment may facilitate more effective penetration of both drugs.[27,28] A 2% sodium chloride solution has been effective for its sclerotic function on scars and adhesions, while a 2% acetic acid solution has been used for decreasing calcific deposits.[29,30] Drugs used for iontophoresis must be water-soluble and ionized. Commercially available drugs manufactured by reputable pharmaceutical companies are recommended. Any medications used for iontophoresis should be manufactured to the standards set forth in the U.S. Pharmacopeia (USP) as they will contain the correct stabilizers and preservatives insuring potency and stability until the drug's expiration date. All medication should be discarded by the expiration date on the drug's label. Any questions regarding the medications used, their indications and contraindications, should be discussed with the physician or pharmacist before use.

Reviewing electrode manufacturer's recommendations for medication use specific to their electrodes should also be done before using iontophoresis. Medications used must be compatible with the material chosen by the manufacturer for the conductive element. Some combinations of drugs and the elements in the reservoir pad may produce undesirable results and outcomes.

Indications

As with any therapeutic intervention, the therapist should be well versed in the pathology and physiology of the patient's condition. Understanding what physiological reaction is needed will assist in identifying which medication and ion to use. Therapists should remain current with the changes in medications, precautions and contraindications of the medications selected, and should periodically review product information and new research before applying iontophoresis or any modality. Each patient will bring a unique perspective to the pathology and should be carefully evaluated to determine optimal treatment goals and therapeutic parameters. Selection of the correct ion and the corresponding polarity is vital to obtaining effective outcomes.

Iontophoresis has been shown to be effective for a variety of disorders based in part on the practice emphasis of the researcher or clinician. Dentists have used iontophoresis for tempero-mandibular joint disease (TMJ), ENT's have used a 2% copper solution for treating allergic rhinitis, and a 20% zinc oxide ointment has been used to facilitate healing for otitis, dermatitis, ulcerations, and open lesions. The most frequent use of iontophoresis in physical medicine and rehabilitation is for inflammation and for local anesthesia.

Inflammatory Conditions

Iontophoresis is widely used and indicated in the treatment of localized inflammation. Delivery of water-soluble corticosteroids can be used for many of the inflammatory conditions affecting joints and soft tissue. Iontophoresis can be used for inflammatory conditions of the extremities, spine, or the TMJ. The most commonly used medication for treating inflammatory conditions using iontophoresis is a 0.4% dexamethasone sodium phosphate with the drug electrode polarity being negative. The dispersive pad polarity should be positive with the recommended dosage for patients with sensitive skin being 2mA x 12 minutes = 24 mA-minutes for a small electrode such as the TransQ which holds 1.5 cc of corticosteroid in the reservoir.

For a local anesthetic effect, many therapists use a 4% lidocaine hydrochloride solution. The lidocaine provides a local anesthetic effect for immediate pain relief. The amount of medication drawn up and placed into the electrode is dependent on the size of the drug electrode. A small TransQ drug electrode holds 1.5 cc of medication with the drug electrode polarity being positive, the dispersive pad polarity being negative. The recommended dosage is 40mA/min.

Some therapists will want to combine the two medications for the benefits of both the anesthetic effect and the anti-inflammatory benefits. The medications utilized would be the corticosteroid (0.4% for injection, USP) combined with the local anesthetic of 4.0%. For treatment with both medications, the drug electrode polarity would be negative, with the therapist alternating the polarity of the drug electrode to positive to ensure greatest absorption of both medications. When combining drugs for delivery in iontophoresis, one drug will most often be delivered more effectively than the other and the concentrations of the medications should be adjusted. To achieve an equal dose of a large and small drug, the concentration of the larger, less mobile drug should be increased.[31]

Discussing the medications and their chemical components with the pharmacist helps to ensure the safety, currency, and efficacy of the medication and the treatment. As most pharmacists dispense IV solutions used for iontophoresis, commercially available products from reputable companies should be used to ensure their purity, concentration, stability and potential interactions.[32,33] Patients should always be questioned as to any known allergies, reactions or sensitivities to foods or medications. Patients have been known to have a variety of reactions to medications including anaphylaxis which can be life threatening, is considered a medical emergency, and should be responded to immediately.

Though most often safe and effective, therapists need to recognize that they are introducing potent medications into the patient, and utmost care should and precautions should be taken. Documented orders from the patient's physician for iontophoresis should always be obtained prior to using iontophoresis, and any questions or concerns should be directed to the referring physician.

Guide to Application

As with any therapeutic intervention, informing the patient is primary. Properly positioning the patient is important, and the patient should never lie on an electrode, as the area being treated may burn. The therapist should prepare the skin surface by trimming any excess hair with scissors to ensure proper adhesion of the electrodes. Electrode sites should never be shaved. Use of creams, gels or other modalities prior to iontophoresis may cause skin irritation and limit drug penetration (Figure 8-1).

1. Hydrate the drug electrode. Use water-soluble 4 mg/ml, or 0.4% corticosteroid, frequently labeled "...for injection, U.S.P". It is important that the drug electrode be sufficiently filled to avoid dry spots which may cause some of the units such as the Dupel to shut down or it may cause skin irritation under the electrode.

2. Prepare the electrode sites by cleaning the areas vigorously with alcohol, allowing the skin to dry completely. Do not apply the electrodes if the skin is irritated; apply only on intact skin. Therapists should note the dryness of the skin, excessively oily skin and the humidity, all of which can influence the resistance of the skin and the effectiveness of the drug delivery.

3. Apply the electrodes. Place the drug electrode on the primary site to be treated. The dispersive electrode should be placed over a major muscle approximately 4-6 inches away from the medicated electrode. Binding or compressing the electrodes by using tape or weights should be avoided during treatment.

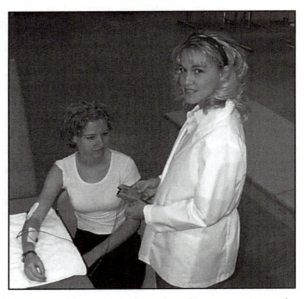

Figure 8-1. Iontophoresis application. Medicated electrode is placed over the targeted tissue.

4. Connect the lead clips to the electrodes. Make sure that the clips are oriented appropriately and keep the clips clean and dry. Avoid pulling on the leads during the treatment and when removing the clips from the electrodes.

5. Begin the treatment. Set the parameters, dependent on the equipment being used. Set the time, set the current, slowly ramping the current up to patient tolerance. Using a lower dosage reduces the chances of skin irritation. Have the patient remain still throughout the session. Most of the equipment available today has dual channels, so the therapist can effectively target two areas for iontophoresis if necessary.

6. After the treatment, a soothing lotion which is non-irritating and has a neutral pH such as aloe vera gel should be applied to the area. The patient should be well instructed in appropriate skin care, and the therapist should note any erythema or skin breakdown which may occur. If the skin is not intact or lesions develop, iontophoresis should be discontinued or the frequency decreased.[34]

Precautions and Contraindications

Patients with known sensitivity or allergy to the medications being administered should never have iontophoresis. The potential for an anaphylactic reaction can be great. Contraindications for the specific medications being used should also be researched by the therapist. Therapists should make sure to discuss with the pharmacist the medications being prescribed by the physician and any related questions. Confirmation of the treatment protocol should be confirmed with the physician. Therapists should refer to the *Physicians Desk Reference*, and should read and keep on file the brochure which comes with each medication.

Care should be used with patients who are pregnant or may be pregnant, as the safety and effectiveness of some medications has not been adequately established. It is better to err on the side of caution! Patients with diabetes who are insulin dependent may notice fluctuations in their blood sugar levels after treatment with corticosteroids. Care should be used when working with diabetic patients who are poorly controlled.

Table 8-1. Commonly Used Ions for Iontophoresis

Medication	Therapeutic Indications	Polarity
Lidocaine hydrochloride	Analgesia; bursitis, neuritis	+
1% & 2% Sodium salicylate	Analgesia; plantar warts	-
Hyaluronidase (Wydase)	Swelling; sprains, strains	+
Tap water	Hyperhidrosis of palms/feet	+/-
2% Copper sulfate	Antibacterial, fungicidal; athlete's foot	+
2% Acetic Acid solution	Calcium deposits, calcific tendonitis myositis, ossificans; musculoskeletal conditions	-
1mL 0.4% Decadron Dexamethasone sodium phosphate	Antiinflammatory, osteoarthritis, bursitis, tendonitis	-

Patients should always be asked if they have any known food allergies or sensitivities, particularly those sensitive to sulfites, which are a preservative. Patients with allergies to shellfish may also react to Iodex, which is used for scar management.

Summary

Iontophoresis is the application of direct electrical current to enhance drug delivery of ionic drugs from aqueous solutions. Iontophoresis provides a localized concentration of a medication to the tissue while avoiding the difficulties of systemic effects. Iontophoresis can be safely and effectively used with patients who are fearful of the pain associated with intramuscular needle injections. Benefits of iontophoresing medications into specific tissues include the fact that the medication can be delivered to a larger area than for an injection. Using iontophoresis in conjunction with traditional modalities and interventions may provide quicker reduction in patient symptoms thereby facilitating occupational function.[35] Additionally, the treatment is repeatable, which allows for a longer period of therapeutic exposure to the medication, thereby facilitating therapeutic benefits and outcomes (Table 8-1).

Case Study

TS is a 41 y/o dental assistant with a diagnosis of right lateral epicondylitis. The patient has been taking nonsteroidal antiinflammatory drugs for the past 6 weeks before being referred to occupational therapy. The patient reports that the medication has provided mild relief, but her symptoms of pain following work or homemaking tasks has continued. The patient reports that she is now having pain and discomfort at rest, and when she rolls onto the arm when sleeping. She relates that symptoms are less severe after waking; but that she "hurts more" as the day progresses. She rates her pain during activities at a 7/10, with the pain described as a "toothache" in the arm. She does have numbness and tingling in the hand with overuse. She has had increasing difficulty manipulating the equipment at the office. Her occupational tasks at work require her to use both hands to assist the dentist. She spends much of the day reaching across the patient or with her arms fully extended, reaching and transferring tools and materials. She has begun to use her nondominant left hand since she is worried that she will drop something while assisting.

Assessment reveals intact skin integrity with the posterior forearm warmer to the touch with a "boggy" feeling. Circumferential measurements reveal a 7-centimeter increase over the nondominant extremity. This discrepancy may be due to increased muscle bulk of the dominant arm, but wrist and mcp measurements are minimally different. ROM measurements reveal wrist flexion 0-55 degrees, wrist extension, 0-50 degrees. Pronation is within normal limits (WNLs) with supination 0-70 degrees. Finger, elbow, and shoulder ROMs are all WNL. Muscle strength is 4/5 with pain on resisted wrist extension. Grip strength on the left is 80#, 45# on the right. There are also noticeable differences in pinch strengths between the dominant and nondominant hand. She exhibits increased pain, with palpation along the lateral epicondyle and the radiohumeral joint. Joint distraction and anterior-posterior glides are restricted.

The patient's signs and symptoms are consistent with lateral epicondylitis, with point tenderness over the extensor tendon origin, pain with wrist loading in extension and limited wrist movement. The patient is educated in work modification and joint protection techniques; including a HEP requiring icing of the elbow as needed after her patients. She is provided with a soft wrist splint for the right and instructed to wear during the day when manipulating objects or when in a static position. Treatment plans include ice massage, and iontophoresis using 0.4% dexamethasone sodium phosphate with the drug delivery electrode placed over the area of point tenderness. Iontophoresis was used to decrease the inflammation and was used as a component of the treatment protocol including stretching exercises and joint mobilization. When the inflammation was decreased and the symptoms abated, involvement in occupational activities simulating the work related movements were implemented to strengthen the weakened muscles and to problem solve possible ergonomic adaptations and movements.

References

1. Banga AK, Chien YW. Iontophoretic delivery of drugs: fundamentals, developments and biomedical applications. *J Contr Release*. 1998;1.

2. Glass JM, Stephen RL, Jacobson SC. The quantity and distribution of radiolabeled dexamethasone delivered to tissue by iontophoresis: *International Journal of Dermatology*. 1980;19(9): 519-524.

3. Singh P, Mailbach HI. Topical iontophoretic drug delivery in vivo: historical development, devices and future perspectives. *Dermatology*. 1993;187, 235-238.

4. LeDuc S, MacKenna RW (translator). *Electric Ions and Their Use in Medicine.* London: Rebman Ltd; 1908.

5. Christopher E, Schebert C, Goos M, The Epidermis. In: Greaves MW, Shester S, eds. *Pharmacology of the Skin I*, Berlin: Springer-Verlag; 1989.

6. Singh J, Roberts MS. Transdermal delivery of drugs by iontophoresis: a review. *Drug Design Deliv.* 1989;4:1.

7. Busby A. Dexamethasone use in iontophoresis, *Sports Medicine.* 1990:10,2.

8. Cullander C. What are the pathways of iontophoretic current flow through mammalian skin? *Adv Drug Del.* 1992;9:119.

9. Cummings J. Iontophoresis. In: Nelson RM and Currier DP, eds. *Clinical Electrotherapy.* Stamford, CT: Appleton and Lange, 1987;231-241.

10. Stilwell GK. Electrotherapy. In: Kottle F, Stillwell G, Lehman J, eds. *Handbook of Physical Medicine and Rehabilitation.* Philadelphia, Pa: W.B. Saunders, 1982;370.

11. Kahn J. *Principles and Practice of Electrotherapy.* 3rd ed. London, Churchill Livingstone. 1995.

12. Hasson SH. Exercise training and dexamethasone iontophoresis in rheumatoid arthritis: A case study. *Physiotherapy.* Canada, 1991;43;11.

13. Glass JM, Stephen RL, Jacobson SC. The quantity and distribution of radiolabeled dexamethasone delivered to tissue by iontophoresis. *Int J Dermatol.* 1980;19:519.

14. Yoshida NY, Roberts MS. Structure transport relationships in transdermal iontophoresis. *Adv Drug Del Dev.* 1992;9:230.

15. Personal correspondence, EMPI Company, April, 1999.

16. Harris P. Iontophoresis: Clinical research in musculoskeletal inflammatory conditions. *Journal of Orthop & Sports Phys Ther.* 1982;4:109-110.

17. Puig CJ, Haenschen RJ, Clark RN. Iontophoretic anesthesia in hair transplantation. *Intl Journ of Aesthetic and Restorative Surgery.* 1993;1:9-12.

18. Maloney M, Bezzant J, Petelenz T. Iontophoretic administration of lidocaine anesthesia in office practice, an appraisal. *Journal of Dermatologic Surgery and Oncology.* 1992;18:937-940.

19. Tamburrini LR, DiMonte M, Sfreddo P. Iontophoresis of corticosteroids in senile osteo arthropathy treatment. *J Gerontol Abstract.* no. 4. 1987.

20. Banta CA. A prospective non-randomized study of iontophoresis. *J Occup Med.* 1994; 36:166.

21. Bertolucci LE. Introduction of anti-inflammatory drugs by iontophoresis: double-blind study. *J Orthop Sports Phys Ther.* 1982;4:103.

22. Harris PR. Iontophoresis: clinical research in musculoskeletal inflammatory conditions. *J Orthop Sports Phys Ther.* 1982;4:109.

23. Tannenbaum M. Iodine iontophoresis in reducing scar tissue. *J Phys Ther.* 1980;60:792.

24. Russo J Jr, Lipman AG, Page BC, Stephen RL. Lidocaine anaesthesia: Comparison of iontophoresis, injection and swabbing. *Am J Hosp Pharm.* 37(6):843-7, 1980.

25. Echols DF, Norris CH, Tabb HG. Anaesthesia of the arc by iontophoresis of lidocaine. *Arch Otolaryngol.* 1975;101:418.

26. Elgart ML, Fuchs G. Tapwater iontophoresis in the treatment of hyperhydrosis. *Int. J Dermatol.* 1987;26:194.

27. Bogner R, Banga A. Iontophoresis and phonophoresis. *U.S. Pharmacist.* 1994;8:14.

28. Petelenz TJ, Buttke JA, Bonds C. Iontophoresis of dexamethasone: laboratory Studies, *J Cont Rel.* 1992;20, 55-66.

29. Kahn J. Acetic acid iontophoresis for calcium deposits. *JAPTA.* 1977;57:658.

30. Kahn J. *Iontophoresis in Principles and Practice of Electrotherapy.* New York: Churchill Livingstone; 1994:136.

31. Banga A, Chien YW. Iontophoretic delivery of drugs: Fundamentals, developments and biomedical applications. *J. Cont. Rel.* 1988;7 ,1-24.

32. *Selected performance characteristics of different iontophoretic electrodes.* Iomed, Inc., and Center of Engineering Design, U. of Utah, 1989.

33. Gangarosa L, Park N, Fong B, et al. Conductivity of drugs used for iontophoresis. *J. Pharm Sci.* 1978; 67:1439-1433.

34. *Phoresor application guide.* Iomed, Inc. 1994.

35. Gudeman SD, Eisele SA, Heidt RS. Treatment of plantar fasciitis by iontophoresis of 0.4% dexamethasone, A randomized, double-blind, placebo-controlled study. *Am Journal of Sports Med.* 1997;25:3, 312-316.

Chapter Nine

Principles of Electrotherapy

Learning Objectives

1. Describe the principles and concepts of electricity.
2. Describe the forms of electrical stimulation and their characteristics.
3. Identify the physiological effects of electrical stimulation on the body.
4. Define and discuss stimulation parameters.
5. Discuss the types and selection of electrodes and their placement.

Terminology

Action Potential	Electrode	Phase Duration
Alternating Current (AC)	EMS	Polyphasic
Biphasic	ESTR	Propagation
Capacitance	FES	Pulsatile Current
Conductance	Frequency	Pulse Duration
Decay Time	Impedance	Reactance
Depolarization	Modulation	Resistance
Direct Current(DC)	Monophasic	Rise Time
Duty Cycle	NMES	Wave Form

Background

The use of electric current to stimulate muscle contraction has a long and colorful history dating as far back as 48 AD, when Scribonius Largus, a Roman physician, used torpedo fish in the treatment of chronic headache and gout. In the late 1700s, Luigi Galvani first noted a frog's legs jumping when stimulated by static electric charges from lightening conducted through his copper down spouts and railings. Through the years there have been numerous claims of medical cures attributed to electricity. Some were propagated by the charlatans and snake oil salesmen of the time. Others have had a more thorough grounding in science and research. These have led to some of the more contemporary applications of electricity in medicine and therapy. Some of these include Kratzenstein, who reported the use of electrification to treat a paralyzed limb. Seiler reported treating scoliosis patients, and Deluc pioneered the concept of ion transfer, or iontophoresis.[1-3]

Growth in the use of electrical stimulation has accelerated since 1965, in part due to the research of Melzack and Wall and their Gate Theory of pain along with advances in technology. Manufacturers continue to develop smaller, more portable units with greater options for the clinician and easier use for patients in their home. In order to understand the therapeutic application of electrical stimulation, the therapist must have a basic knowledge of the terminology and principles.

There are a number of clinical methods for applying electrical stimuli to patients in order to accomplish a variety of therapeutic purposes. Terminology for specific applications is based in part on the therapeutic goals. Frequently used applications of electrical stimulation include: electrical muscle stimulation (EMS) for stimulation of denervated muscle; neuromuscular electrical stimulation (NMES) for stimulation of innervated muscle; functional electrical stimulation (FES); electrical stimulation for tissue repair (ESTR); and transcutaneous electrical nerve stimulation (TENS). Common terms used include: NMES, TENS, High Voltage Galvanic, and Iontophoresis.[4]

NMES is the use of electrical stimulation to activate muscles through the stimulation of the intact peripheral nerve, achieving a motor response. FES and functional neuromuscular stimulation (FNS) are forms of NMES and are used as a substitute for orthotics to assist in functional activities such as grasping an object. NMES uses a pulsating alternating current (AC) and is used for the stimulation of innervated tissues. NMES is often used to reduce muscle spasm, for muscle strengthening, and for edema reduction which occurs through muscle pumping action.

TENS is a generic term used to describe a class of stimulator used for pain control. Although the term TENS actually encompasses all forms of electrical stimulation, it has become synonymous with pain control over the last several years. TENS also uses surface electrodes delivering the stimulation across the skin, with the treatment goal being sensory analgesia rather than motor response.

High voltage galvanic stimulation, or electrical stimulation for tissue repair (ESTR) refers to a class of stimulator that uses an interrupted monophasic wave form greater than 100 volts. Electrical stimulation for tissue repair has been used in the treatment of chronic and acute edema, chronic and acute pain, wound healing, muscle spasm, delaying atrophy, and increasing blood flow.

Iontophoresis is the induction of topically applied ions into the tissue by application of a low-voltage direct galvanic current. Iontophoresis is typically used for treatment of inflammatory conditions such as tendinitis, and for scar formation.

The therapeutic current used in treatment and the characteristics of the current will determine the clinical application. Neuromuscular electrical stimulation can be used for muscle reeducation, reduction of spasticity, delay of atrophy, and muscle strengthening.

Basic Electrical Principles

Electrical current is the flow or movement of ions or electrons, charged particles, from one point to another in order to equalize the charge. Electricity is a type of energy which exhibits magnetic, chemical, mechanical, and thermal effects. Electrical current occurs when there is an imbalance in the number of electrons in two locations. Current most often takes the path of least resistance and flows from an area of high electron concentration (cathode) to an area with less concentration, the anode or "positive pole". There are three primary forms of electrical current used in clinical application: direct current (DC), alternating current (AC), and pulsatile (pulsed) current (PC).[4]

Electrical Stimulation Forms

Direct Current

DC is unidirectional and occurs when the electrons flow continuously in one direction. DC has often been termed "galvanic current" to describe the uninterrupted, unidirectional flow of charged particles. The direction of the current flow, from a negative electrode to a positive electrode, or vice versa, can be selected depending on the electrical stimulation equipment being used. The electrodes maintain their polarity. The basic pattern used to characterize DC flow is the square wave characterized by the current flowing continuously until the circuit is disconnected or the battery is turned off.[5] Use of DC can cause chemical reactions in the body: tissues with acidic reactions occurring at the anode due to oxidation of the anions, alkaline reactions can occur at the cathode. DC is used to facilitate the ionization of medication through the skin (iontophoresis) and can also be used to stimulate denervated muscle.[6]

Alternating Current

AC is a type of current that periodically changes its direction of flow. The current flow remains uninterrupted, but it is bidirectional. The charged particles change directions and there is no true positive or negative pole. The electrical fields alternate and change polarity. Household electricity uses AC. The terms biphasic waveform and bidirectional current have also been used to describe AC. Because the electrodes are changing their polarity with the shift in the direction of the current, there are minimal chemical effects to the tissue. Hertz (Hz) is the term used to measure the number of times that the current reverses direction in one second (cycles per second). A current of 1 megahertz (MHz) would change the direction of current one million times per second.

Pulsatile Current

The term *pulsed current* has also been used to describe modifications to the current, whereby the electron flow is periodically interrupted (Figure 9-1). Pulsed current can

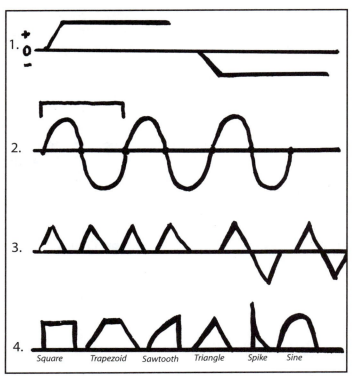

Figure 9-1. Types of current. 1) Direct current. 2) Alternating current. 3) Pulsatile current. 4) Classifiers of interrupted direct current, one phase of AC, or one phase of a pulse. illustration by Kim Bartlett. Used with permission.

flow in an unidirectional (monophasic) or bi-directional (biphasic) movement. The current is interrupted for extremely short periods of time—milliseconds or microseconds. Essentially the current is being turned on and off in a rapid fashion and can be visualized best if one thinks of a strobe light, flashing on and off. The current, in effect, is pulsed over time and the reaction on the tissue is dependent on whether the parameters are set for unidirectional effect or bidirectional effect.[7] There are a number of pulses with varying shapes or waveforms (pulse types) which have been used clinically and have led to some confusion among clinicians. Pulsatile current is the most frequently used current form in the clinic. Most stimulators can be classified under one of three waveforms: monophasic, biphasic, or polyphasic.

The geometric or visual representation of an electrical current flow or stimulus is known as the waveform. The geometric shape of the wave describes the amplitude and the pulse duration of each stimulus. The basic properties of the electrical current flow are the amplitude (or intensity) and the duration (or length) of the current. The isoelectric point is the level which sets the baseline where the electrical potential between the two poles is considered equal, or zero, with no current flow. The amplitude is the level or distance that the impulse rises above or below the baseline. The pulse duration is the horizontal or lateral distance or length which is required to complete the shape of the electrical flow. Pulse width has been used in the past for pulse duration but standardization of terminology precludes its use. The complete area within the waveform represents the total current that the pulse contains.[8]

Monophasic

This waveform has one phase to a single pulse with a unidirectional current flow. Current flow is in one direction and may possess either negative or positive polarity (Figure 9-2).

Figure 9-2. Pulsatile waveform classifications: monophasic, biphasic and polyphasic. Biphasic waveforms can be symmetrical or asymmetrical, and balanced or unbalanced. Illustration by Kim Bartlett. Used with permission.

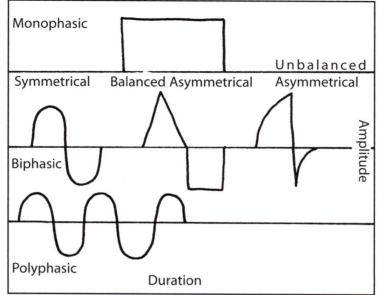

Biphasic

Biphasic currents possess two opposing phases which are contained in a single pulse. This pulse is bidirectional with the lead phase of the pulse above the baseline and the final phase below the baseline. A symmetrical biphasic pulse occurs when the two phases deviate from the baseline in an identical and equal manner, one phase in a positive direction and the succeeding phase in the negative direction. The two phases of the pulse are equal in magnitude and duration and therefore the charges of the two phases cancel each other out and the pulse is balanced.

A pulse becomes asymmetrical biphasic when the two phases are not identical. If the electrical charges of both phases are equal, the pulse is considered balanced and the charges will cancel each other out. This is known as a zero net charge (ZNC). If the electrical charge in one phase is greater than the other phase, the net charge across the baseline produces residual physiological changes due to the change in polarity. This type of pulse is described as an unbalanced asymmetrical biphasic (Figure 9-3). Many of the commercial neuromuscular units and TENS units are capable of producing both balanced and unbalanced asymmetrical biphasic waveforms, however, the symmetrical biphasic waveforms are more comfortable for the patient due to the lower charges per phase.

Polyphasic

Polyphasic waveforms consist of a burst of three or more phases. A burst consists of a series of pulses which are delivered as a single charge. This type of current has been known as interferential current and "Russian" current. Though there have been many claims that this type of current is unique, there are no known physiologic advantages to using this type of waveform. Physiologically, the body perceives the burst as a single pulse. The burst can be monophasic or biphasic and contain a single charge.

Figure 9-3. A. Peak amplitude B. Peak to peak amplitude. Illustration by Kim Bartlett. Used with permission.

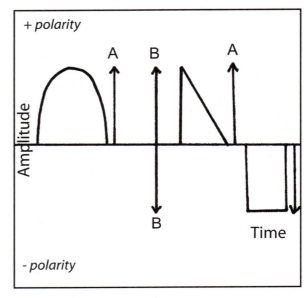

Figure 9-4. A. Phase duration B. Pulse duration. C. Peak to peak amplitude. Illustration by Kim Bartlett. Used with permission.

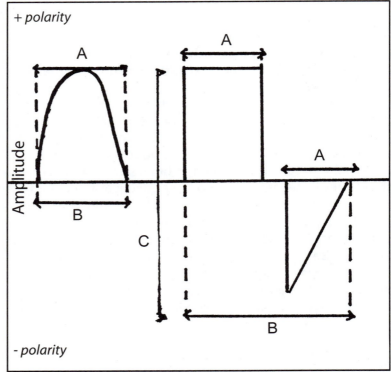

General Characteristics of the Waveform (Pulse)

The clinician has a wide selection of electrical stimulators to choose from. Selecting the appropriate equipment is based in part on the treatment goal, the equipment available, and the patient's preference, or perceived comfort, of the waveform. Though patient compliance and comfort will vary, the symmetrical biphasic waveform appears to provide the highest tolerance and comfort level.[9-11] The geometric representation of the electrical pulse or stimulus is referred to as the waveform.[12] There are three primary characteristics of the waveform, the amplitude, duration, and the rate of onset.

Amplitude

The maximum amount of current or voltage which occurs during one phase of a pulse is known as the peak amplitude (Figure 9-4). Increasing the amplitude increases the charge of the pulse. Average current is the total current per unit of time and is determined by averaging the current amplitude over the duration or length of the waveform. Milliamperes or microamperes are the measurement used to describe the peak amplitude in current though some equipment also uses voltage (volts). Amplitude is frequently labeled or termed *intensity*. The peak amplitude measures the magnitude of the stimulus during a monophasic pulse, and measures the amplitude from the zero line to the maximum positive or negative point. Peak to peak amplitude is measured from the positive most point to the negative most point which occurs during the two phases of biphasic pulse, or the two phases of one cycle of AC.

Resistance

Resistance is the property of a substance which opposes or resists the flow of current. The unit of resistance is the ohm, and the amount of resistance of a given material is determined by Ohm's law. The greater the resistance or "impedance" in an electrical circuit, the lower the rate of electrical flow. Current flow is directly proportional to voltage. If there is an increase in voltage combined with constant resistance, the current increases. Current flow is also inversely related to resistance. If there is an increase in resistance combined with constant voltage, current decreases. Ohm's law accounts for the relationship between amperage, voltage, and resistance, and can be shown by the following equations:

$$I = V/R \quad \text{or} \quad V = IR$$

"I" is the current intensity in amperes, "V" is the potential difference in volts, and "R" is the resistance in ohms. The voltage (V) must be sufficient to overcome the resistance for the current (I) to exist. Clinically, this concept is important since high skin impedance necessitates a high voltage to allow the current to flow into the tissue below.[13,14] The ability of a material to conduct a current rather than resist the current is known as conductance and is considered the inverse of resistance.

Characteristics of Electricity and Physiological Implications

The ability to store a charge in an electric field and oppose change in the current flow is termed capacitance. Nerve and muscle membranes serve as capacitors, while the nerve-muscle complex functions as the conductors. Conversely, skin and adipose tissue function as insulators, and resist current flow. Conductance is the ease with which the current moves, and in the body is dependent, in part, on the water content of the tissue. Tissue with a low water content is less conductive. Nerve and muscle components display higher water contents though the membranes provide a high degree of reactance. Skin is also a factor, as the amount of moisture within the skin will impede the flow of current, particularly if the skin is dry. Skin provides the greatest resistive element to the flow of the current since it contains very little fluid. Increasing the moisture of the skin through heat, which also increases the surface salt content, facilitates conductivity of the current.[13,14]

Impedance is the opposition of the current flow in tissue and can be visualized as the "resistance" to the current. Impedance consists of the properties of resistance and reactance. Reactance is also termed capacitive resistance and is the result of counter-voltage which occurs due to electrolytic polarization when current is conducted through the tissues. Ions accumulate at the tissue interface and cell membrane creating a charge opposite to that of the voltage being applied at the electrode. This counter-voltage is called reactance or capacitive resistance.

Electrical Stimulation Parameters

Depth of Penetration

Stimulators on the market today can be classified as high- or low-voltage. A unit which uses a high-voltage output is capable of producing a high peak amplitude. Low-voltage units are those in the range of one to 100 volts. High-voltage units have an output of 500 volts. There is a relationship between the peak amplitude and the depth of the electrical current penetration. If the biological tissue which is to be stimulated is similar, the higher the voltage applied, the larger the current that will be passed through the tissue. Low-voltage stimulation delivers less current through the tissue. The conductivity of the tissue being stimulated will determine how deep the penetration will be.[15] Tissue such as bone, fat, or adipose tissue conduct current poorly and will limit the depth of penetration of the voltage.

Duration

Pulse duration is the time period from the beginning of the phase to the conclusion of the final phase including the intrapulse interval. Phase duration refers to the length of time between the beginning and the end of one phase of the pulse. In a monophasic current, the phase and pulse duration are synonymous terms. In a biphasic current, the pulse duration is equal to the total of the two-phase durations, including the intrapulse interval.

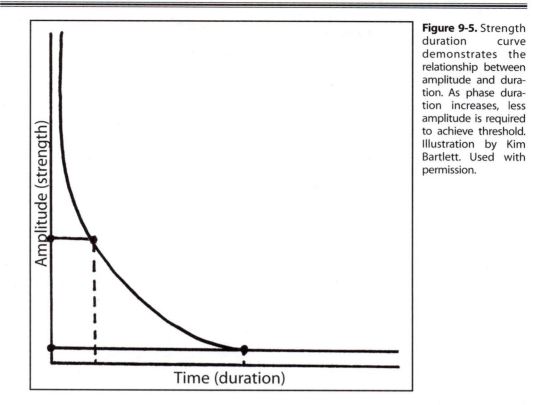

Figure 9-5. Strength duration curve demonstrates the relationship between amplitude and duration. As phase duration increases, less amplitude is required to achieve threshold. Illustration by Kim Bartlett. Used with permission.

The phase duration is a vital factor in determining which type of tissue will be stimulated and the comfort of the stimulation. As the phase duration increases, the comfort level decreases. There is also a direct effect to the degree of chemical changes occurring in the tissue and the phase duration, increased durations cause an increase in chemical effects. A shorter pulse and a short phase duration result in better conductivity of the current into the tissue with less impedance[16] (Figure 9-5).

Rise Time and Decay Time

Rise time and decay times are associated with their pulse shapes. The amount of time that is needed for the amplitude (wave form) to go from zero volts to its peak is known as the rise time. The rate of the rise can cause a rapid nerve depolarization. The rate of the rise is directly related to the ability of the amplitude to excite nervous tissue. If the rise is slow, the nerve membrane can accommodate or adjust to the voltage change and an action potential may not be reached. Rise times occur very quickly and are measured in nanoseconds (Ns), which is one billionth of a second, or up to several hundred milliseconds (ms), thousands of a second, or they may be longer. The amount of time it takes for the peak amplitude to return back to zero volts from its peak is known as the decay time (Figure 9-6).

Frequency

The number of pulses, or wave forms, which are repeated at regular intervals is known as the pulse frequency.[17] The pulse frequency is referred to as pulses per second (pps) and consists of the number of pulses (or cycles) per second delivered to the body.

Figure 9-6. A. Peak Amplitude. B. Rise Time. C. Decay Time. D. Intrapulse Interval. Illustration by Kim Bartlett. Used with permission.

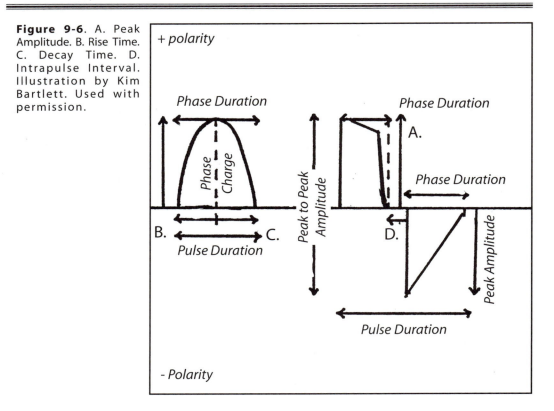

The frequency of the stimuli output is also known as the *carrier* frequency. The carrier frequency is the base frequency of the AC sine wave and is described in hertz (Hz) or cycles per seconds (cps). The carrier frequency consists of three primary classifications: low-frequency currents (<1000 Hz); medium-frequency currents (1000-10000 Hz); high-frequency current (>10000 Hz). For the most part, most therapeutic electrical stimulation devices are low frequency. Some manufacturers have developed equipment that uses an AC carrier frequency which administers a low-frequency current as an electrical burst and has added to the confusion. This burst is a series of cycles that results in depolarization of the sensory and motor nerves.[18]

On most of the equipment available for electrical stimulation, the frequency may be adjusted and may be labeled pulse rate. There is an inverse relationship between the pulse frequency of the current and the capacitive resistance of the tissue; a low pps encounters greater tissue resistance than current with a higher pps with an increase in the intensity needed to accommodate the resistance. Impedance decreases as the frequency increases. A frequency range of one to 120 pps being effective for most therapeutic purposes and will be the most comfortable.[19,20]

Duty Cycle

The duty cycle refers to the amount of time between the stimulation period and the rest period. Other terms frequently used to describe this concept include the on/off cycle, or reciprocate. The on time consists of the length of time that the current is being delivered to the patient. The off time is the period of time when the current has been stopped. The duty cycle is often expressed as a percentage, or ratio. For example, a current which is on for 5 seconds and off for 20 seconds would have a ratio of 1:4. To express the duty cycle as a percentage, one divides the time the current is on by the total cycle time (consists of the time the current is on plus the off time). Using the previous on time (5 seconds) and off time (20 seconds), the equation would be:

$$\frac{\text{On Time (5 seconds)}}{\text{On Time (5 seconds) + Off Time (20 seconds)}} \times 100$$

$$= \frac{5 \text{ seconds (On Time)}}{25 \text{ seconds (Total Cycle Time)}} \times 100$$

$$= 0.2 \times 100$$

$$= 20\% \text{ duty cycle}$$

The duty cycle is critical in order to be able to calculate the total stimulation time and is important in determining the amount of potential muscle fatigue. As the patient's condition improves, the duty cycle can be progressively increased. If the off time is longer than the on time, less muscle fatigue will occur[21] (See Figure 9-6).

Current Modulation, Ramp Time

Changes made in the applied current or to the pulse characteristics are referred to as modulation. The pulse or current can be modified by changes in the frequency, amplitude and duration. These parameters can be modified individually, intermittently, or sequentially, and alter the quality of the response. Forms of current modulation include interruption of the current or ramping of the current. Ramping is a change of the pulse intensity or duration. When the current is increasing to the maximum peak it is ramping up, when it is decreasing it is ramping down (Figure 9-7).

Ramp time refers to the length of time it takes for the current to go from zero to peak amplitude. The current intensity will gradually increase over a predetermined period, most often from one to eight seconds. Ramp down refers to the gradual decrease of intensity at the end of the ON time, or the length of time it takes the current to move from its peak amplitude back to zero. The ramp time describes the change in amplitude of the current over a specific time period of the current flow and is different from the rise time which describes amplitude of a single pulse.[22] Some stimulation equipment allows the therapist to adjust the ramp feature though the parameter may be preset. The ramp time affords a degree of comfort of the stimulation, and a two second ramp may be sufficient for the patient. As spasticity increases, the ramp-up should be increased in an attempt to avoid a quick stretch of the spastic muscle by a sudden surge of the stimulus. When determining the total on time for muscle contraction, the ramp-up time should also be added to the equation.

Burst refers to a type of modulation in which a finite series of pulses, or an envelope of alternation current is delivered at a specific frequency or a specific time interval (burst duration). Bursts usually flow for a few milliseconds with a few milliseconds interruption. It should be noted here that a true interrupted current occurs when pulses flow for one second or more and then are interrupted for one second or more. Though there is an abbreviated interruption to the stimulus, bursts do not allow true interruption of muscle contraction. In order to provide adjustable interruption of current to achieve increases in strength, tendon excursion, or edema control, it is important to have interruptions of muscle contraction.

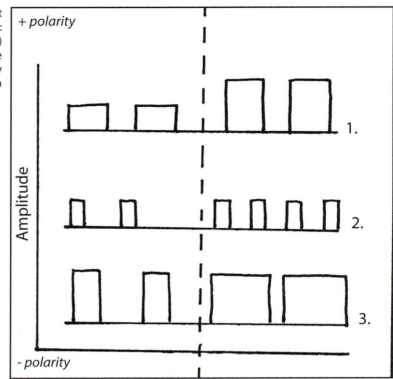

Figure 9-7. Current increased by increasing: 1) Peak amplitude, 2) Pulse frequency, 3) Phase duration. Illustration by Kim Bartlett. Used with permission.

Physiological Basis of Nerve and Muscle Excitation

When electrical current is delivered to tissues, alterations in the physiological process of the tissue can occur at a localized or cellular level, segmentally, and systemically. Electrical current can modify the physiologic response and physiochemical effects of the tissue. Tissues possess unique properties and are considered either excitable or nonexcitable. Nerve and muscles are considered excitable tissues, and their ability to initiate and propagate an action potential is the basis for the therapeutic use of electrotherapeutic interventions. A general review and understanding of the fundamental neurophysiology of nerve and muscle excitation are necessary in order to understand the principles and response of electrical stimulation.

Nerve and muscle cells are considered excitable and have the ability to maintain an electrical potential across the cell membrane as well as to respond with an alteration in the electrical potential. The resting membrane potential for a nerve and muscle cells is between -60 and -90 millivolts (mV). The cell interior is negative in relationship to the exterior and consists of larger amounts of potassium ions with lower levels of sodium ions. There is an unequal ionic distribution across the membrane due to the increased permeability of the membrane and an active sodium pump.

Action potentials occur when a stimulus excites the nerve causing membrane depolarization. The tissue's response and alteration can be caused by thermal, mechanical, chemical, or electrical stimuli. The action potential occurs due to a decrease in the membrane potential with an increase in the permeability to the sodium ions which increases depolarization. The influx of positively charged sodium ions into the cell causes further depolarization of the membrane and facilitates an increased opening of the

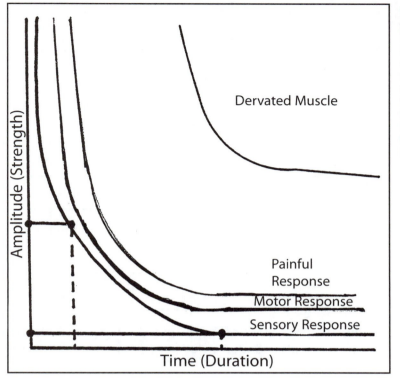

Figure 9-8. Strength—Duration Curve. Relationship between Strength—Duration curves for nerve fibers and denervated skeletal muscles. Less amplitude is needed to reach threshold as time/duration increases. Illustration by Kim Bartlett. Used with permission.

sodium channels. As the sodium ions are flowing into the cell, the potassium ions are exiting from the interior. When an equilibrium potential for sodium is reached, the sodium ion flow slows, and the membrane channels for sodium close. The original diffusion gradient with selective potassium permeability returns and results in a potassium dominated potential again, negative on the inside in comparison to the positive charge outside of the cell. The depolarization of the cell and the stimulation of the action potential takes only 1 to 2 milliseconds.

Action potentials are an all-or-none occurrence; when the threshold of stimulation is reached, the action potential occurs and the cell depolarizes. For the action potential to occur, the stimulus must be of sufficient intensity and duration to cause the ions to move across the membrane. The excitable tissue will respond to the stimulus in the same fashion as it does to an even stronger stimulus. Once the action potential is reached, the potential cannot be graded by changing the intensity or duration of the stimulus. Following the excitation of the tissue, there is a brief period during which the tissue is inexcitable to a second stimulus and cannot be depolarized. This phase is known as the absolute refractory period, and during this time, an action potential cannot occur. The action potential threshold of tissues varies between muscle and nerve fibers with variations occurring among nerve fibers (Figure 9-8).

Propagation

Tissues with higher levels of water content are better able to transmit electricity. Bone, tendon, fascia, and adipose tissue are poor conductors of electrical current due to a low water content. Bone, tendon, fascia, and adipose tissue contain approximately 5-

Table 9-1. Tissue Impedance			
Type of Tissue	**Approximate Water Content**	**Electrical Impedance**	**Electrical Conduction**
bone	5%	highest	poorest
epidermis	10%	higher	poorer
fat	15%	high	poor
muscle	75%	low	good
nerve	80%	lower	better
blood	90%	lowest	best

15% water compared to the 70-90% water content of muscle, nerve, and blood. As noted earlier, the outer layer of skin also conducts electricity poorly due to low water content (Table 9-1).

When an action potential is reached, the excitable membrane can cause an action potential to occur in an adjoining area of the tissue. There is a localized flow of the current around the depolarized site of the action potential which may cause a depolarization in an adjoining area of the membrane. In a nerve or muscle fiber, the action potential can be propagated across the entire membrane following the path of least resistance. Repetitive stimulation can continue to generate action potentials in the tissue. The rate at which the action potential and propagation occur is dependent on the diameter of the fiber and the degree of myelination. Conduction in myelinated fibers is faster than in unmyelinated fibers. Larger diameter fibers also offer less resistance to the conduction current which is generated by the action potential, and conduction occurs faster with temperature elevation. The number of nerve fibers recruited increases as the amplitude and the pulse duration increase. Following an action potential, there is a period of recovery which limits the frequency of the action potentials to occur.

The effect of the electrical current on muscle is dependent on a number of factors including the number of fibers in the motor unit and the amount of stimulation provided by the device. The size of the motor unit varies dependent upon its specific kinesiological function. Some motor units have only a small number of fibers and allow for fine muscle movements. Larger numbers of fibers, 200 or more, up to thousands of muscle fibers are found in large motor units and produce gross motor movement.

The effect of the current on muscle is determined by the amount of stimulation provided by the device. The amplitude/intensity and pulse duration determine the threshold for stimulation of the muscle and the quality of the sensation. The frequency determines the degree of tetany and the rate of fatigue. The duty cycle, which is the on/off time also has an influence on the fatigue level. The rise time affects the rate of accommodation to the electrical stimulus, as well as influencing the spastic/stretch reflex.

Normal Movement and Electrically Stimulated Movement

The adaptation that occurs in response to exercise training is a function of the intensity and the duration of the training stimulus. Facilitating or augmenting muscle strength is based on the overload principle, regardless of whether the muscle contraction is electrically or voluntarily elicited. There is a direct relationship between the training intensity and increase in strength. Stimulation from a motor nerve at the neuromuscular junction serves as the impetus for the muscle action potential causing a contraction.

In normal movement or with a voluntary contraction of a muscle, the motor units fire asynchronously. With a voluntary contraction, the smaller motor units are recruited first with the large motor units recruited as the contraction strength increases. This sequence provides fine motor control with recruitment of the larger fibers occurring when increasing strength is required. This type of recruitment provides for smooth, controlled movement. In electrically stimulated movement, the converse occurs with the large motor units recruited first in a synchronous recruitment pattern. Because of this, the electrically stimulated muscle fatigues more rapidly and lacks the finely controlled quality of movement.

Electrodes and Skin Care

Electrodes act as the interface between the body and the electrical stimulator facilitating the movement of the current through the skin. There are a wide range and variety of electrodes available commercially, and they vary in shape, size and flexibility. The electrode is composed of an electrically conductive material surrounded by a non-conductive material. The type, size, and placement of the electrodes help to determine the effectiveness and ease of treatment. The primary goal is to provide a balanced contraction of the selected muscle group approximating functional movement patterns. Careful selection of electrode size and placement is crucial in obtaining this movement. Correct placement of the electrodes also improves the efficiency of the electrical current and provides for improved patient comfort.

Electrodes are made out of a variety of materials. Electrodes may be metal, carbon-impregnated silicone rubber, or metallic meshed cloth. An interface, or medium, between the electrode and the skin is often needed to decrease skin-electrode resistance. Moistened sponges are frequently used with metal electrodes to decrease the skin-electrode impedance. Carbon-rubber electrodes often use a conducting gel, but sponges and gauze saturated with water often suffice. Sufficient conducting gel should be liberally applied to the entire conducting surface area of the carbon rubber or metal electrodes to decrease the skin-electrode resistance and to improve patient comfort.[23,24]

Electrodes may be self-adhesive, or they may be adhered in place with the use of adhesive patches or tape if nonadhesive electrodes are used. Care must be used to insure complete coverage of the electrode with gel and full contact with the skin. Carbon-impregnated rubber electrodes degrade over time and with prolonged use, and should be replaced as hot spots may develop in the electrode. The hot spot in carbon-rubber electrodes may cause skin irritation, and patients who describe a biting or stinging sensation during electrical stimulation are likely experiencing uneven conductivity. If the patient complains of biting or stinging sensation and discomfort, it is safer to replace the electrode.

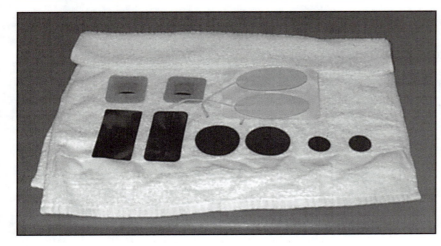

Figure 9-9. Examples of commonly used electrodes for electrotherapy. The black carbon electrodes require the use of gel and can be reused. The lighter-colored electrodes are self-adhering.

Self-adhering electrodes may be reusable and have a foil or metal mesh and a synthetic gel or conductive Karaya covered with an adhesive surface. Because these electrodes do not require strapping or taping, they are very convenient to use, and patient compliance with home programming is increased. Many of these electrodes may be left on for extended periods and are useful for patients on home programs. However, instruction in proper skin care and hygiene is crucial to prevent skin irritation or skin breakdown with prolonged placement of the electrodes. Carbon-rubber electrodes provide the most current at the lowest skin impedance and may be more comfortable for the patient. Resistance of the electrode may indicate the ohms of resistance with larger electrodes having a lower resistance than smaller electrodes (Figure 9-9).

Electrode Size

The smaller the electrode, the higher the current density. There is an inverse relationship between the density of the current and the size of the electrode. As the size of the electrode decreases, the current density increases. If a large electrode is used, the total current is then distributed over a larger surface area. Due to its small surface area, a smaller electrode has a higher current density. Increased current density causes an increased perception of the stimulation under the electrode and a greater physiologic response due to a greater charge transfer. If the current density is too high, it can lead to surface burns and potential tissue damage. It is important to consider the size of the muscles which will be treated when determining electrode size. Size of the stimulated muscle will directly affect the selection of the appropriate size electrode in order to avoid overflow of the current into surrounding tissue which may cause recruitment.

Because of the high current density, smaller electrodes require less current to stimulate the tissue. Larger electrodes produce a stronger contraction with less pain and discomfort. However, the current is spread over a larger area and may affect the physiological response that is desired. Electrode size is determined by the size of the body area which is being treated and the size of the other electrodes being used. The electrode size is determined, in part, by the size of the target tissue. Current density is also greater in the superficial layers of the skin and is less in deeper tissues. Because of this, electrodes should not be placed too closely; placing them further apart results in a deeper penetration of the electrical current.

	Table 9-2. Factors Affecting Electrode Conduction	
a.	Resistance from skin surface due to dirt, sweat, lotions
b.	Areas of excessive adipose tissue
c.	Dry skin, skin irritation, or breakdown
d.	Perspiration residues
e.	Hair (excessive hair can be cut short, cropped close to the skin, avoid shaving the area)
f.	Poor electrode contact with the skin
g.	Electrode spacing (electrodes placed too closely together)

Electrodes are attached to the stimulator through the use of leads or lead wires. Lead wires most often attach to two electrodes by a metal tip that inserts into the electrode. There are a number of different types of electrode-lead wire configurations available such as the pin, pigtail, or snap-to-pin. The tips are prone to corrosion and should be cleaned on a regular basis. Patients who have difficulty with fine motor control or who have poor vision may be more comfortable using the snap-to-pin configuration.

There are a number of factors which may interfere with electrical conduction and increase resistance (Table 9-2).

Electrode Placement

The location and orientation of the electrodes are also a consideration when stimulating muscles. Muscle fibers are more conductive when the current flows with the direction of the muscle fibers, and longitudinal placement may facilitate a stronger contraction. Electrodes can be configured to be monopolar, bipolar, or quadrapolar.

Monopolar Placement

Monopolar techniques involve the use of an active electrode and dispersive electrode.[25] The active electrode is placed over the target area where the treatment effect will occur and is generally smaller in size than the dispersive electrode. The dispersive electrode is used to complete the circuit and is larger, and placed at a distance from the target electrode. Because of the higher current density, the effect of the treatment is concentrated under the active, smaller electrode. Monopolar techniques are used most often for the stimulation of a trigger point or wound healing.[26,27]

Figure 9-10. Dual bipolar electrode placement. Illustration by Kim Bartlett. Used with permission.

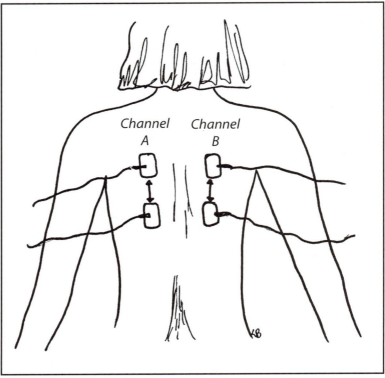

Bipolar Placement

Bipolar techniques require the use of two electrodes from one channel of equal or near-equal size and are located within the target treatment area. Bipolar techniques are most often used for stimulating a large muscle. The patient will perceive an equal amount of stimulation or response under each electrode due to the similar densities. If a motor response is the goal, one electrode should be placed over the motor point, with the other electrode placed elsewhere over the muscle belly. If a larger area is targeted or a combination of movement is required the leads can be bifurcated[28-30] (Figure 9-10).

Quadripolar Placement

Quadripolar techniques use two channels and two sets of electrodes. Essentially, there are four electrodes located within the treatment area and the currents may intersect, intensify, and localize the treatment effect. Quadripolar techniques are often used to stimulate large areas for pain management and in neuromuscular stimulation of antagonistic muscles (Figure 9-11).

Stimulation of Muscle and Nerve Fibers

When stimulating a normal muscle it is not the muscle fiber that is stimulated, but rather the nerve fibers that innervate that muscle. Nerve fibers require a lower intensity and shorter duration of current to evoke a response. Muscle fibers by contrast require a longer pulse duration to achieve the same response. This is clinically important when determining if electric stimulation is indicated and what type to use. In stimulating nerve fibers, thinner, smaller diameter fibers (those usually found in sensory and pain fibers) require higher stimulus intensities with longer duration to achieve a response.

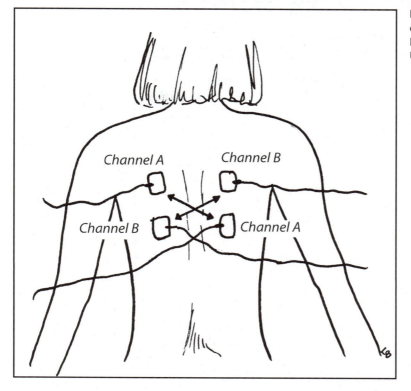

Figure 9-11. Quadrapolar electrode placements. Illustration by Kim Bartlett. Used with permission.

Larger diameter fibers and motor fibers require lower intensity and short duration to achieve a response. When stimulating denervated muscle tissues, it is necessary to stimulate the muscle fiber directly. This will require a long pulse duration such as those found in galvanic or DC currents.[31] Research into treating denervated tissues is somewhat contradictory. One school of thought believes stimulation in the early phases following denervation is necessary to reduce atrophy of muscle fibers and proliferation of fibrous connective tissues in the muscle. To accomplish this, treatment must occur before this process can occur. However, if denervation is expected to be brief and reinervation is expected, stimulation may not be necessary as muscle atrophy and connective tissue formation will not have begun. If denervation is prolonged, and atrophy occurs, stimulation of muscle tissue may be indicated.[32]

In attempting to evoke a motor response in a muscle, it is easier to stimulate the nerve that innervates the muscle directly. There has been a great deal of research over the years advocating the use of electrical stimulation to enhance muscle strength and performance.

In muscle stimulation, NMES has been found to selectively stimulate large, fast twitch muscle fibers. In contrast, traditional exercise will result in first stimulating smaller, slow twitch, type II fibers, then fast twitch fibers. Following injury and immobilization atrophy occurs in the fast twitch, large fibers initially. To achieve similar results of enhancement of large fibers it is necessary to exercise at high intensity, with muscle contractions of 78 to 119% of normal contraction strength.[33,34] This results in an increase in cardiovascular output. If increased heart rate is not a desired response, such as with the elderly and those suffering from cardiovascular disease, NMES may be indicated. If the individual is able to perform exercise at required intensities then NMES may

Table 9-3. Recruitment						
Recruitment Order	Fiber Type and class	Diameter μm	Amplitude	Phase Duration	Pulse/Phase Charge
1st	A Beta	6-12	Lowest	Shortest	Lowest
2nd	A Gamma	2-8			
3rd	A Delta	1-6			
4th	C IV	<1	Highest	Lowest	Highest

not be indicated, as stimulation may not be as effective as exercise. Conversely, NMES may be indicated for a short duration until the individual is able to perform exercise and activities at the required levels[35-38] (Table 9-3).

Physiologic Responses of the Body to Electrical Stimulation

There are specific physiologic responses which can occur at a cellular level, tissue level, or segmentally, within muscle groups during electrical stimulation. The intensity of stimulation is one factor which will determine if the effect enhances or suppresses a specific response. At the cellular level, stimulation may modify fibroblastic and osteoblast activity, facilitate microcirculation, and increase metabolic rate and activity. If the stimulation is of sufficient intensity, there may be skeletal muscle contraction with strengthening or fatigue, smooth muscle contraction or relaxation with its effect on circulation, and influence on tissue regeneration and remodeling. Muscle contraction also has an effect on lymphatic, arterial and venous blood flow. Systemically, there may be a decrease in pain due to the stimulation's effect on neurotransmitters and an increase in endogenous opiates.[39-43] Indications for the use of electrotherapy for innervated muscle tissue, or NMES, include:

1. Range of motion
2. Inhibition of spasticity or muscle spasm
3. Muscle strengthening or disuse atrophy
4. Improving endurance
5. Muscle reeducation or neuromuscular facilitation
6. Orthotic substitution
7. Edema control in both acute and chronic conditions

In denervated muscle, tissue stimulation can be used to maintain muscle integrity, strengthen adjacent muscle groups, or to teach compensatory movements, such as in the case of an incomplete spinal cord injury. Electrical stimulation may also be effective for stimulating tissue repair through improving circulation and/or edema control, facilitate wound healing, and in the transcutaneous delivery of medication, or iontophoresis.[44-52]

References

1. Hunter JM, Mackin E, Callahan AD, eds. *Rehabilitation of the Hand: Surgery and Therapy.* 4th ed. St. Louis, Mo: Mosby, 1995: 1508-1519.

2. Geddes LA. A short history of the electrical stimulation of excitable tissue. *Physiologist* (suppl.) 1984;27:S-1.

3. Licht S. History of electrotherapy. In: Stillwell GK, ed. *Therapeutic Electricity and Ultraviolet Radiation*. 3rd ed. Baltimore/London: Williams & Wilkins; 1983.

4. American Physical Therapy Association. *Electrotherapy Standards Committee of the Section on clinical Electrophysiology of the American Physical Therapy Association: Electrotherapeutic Terminology in Physical Therapy. Section on Clinical Electrophysiology and the American Physical Therapy Association*, Alexandria, 1990.

5. Forster A, Palastanga N. *Clayton's Electrotherapy: Theory and Practice.* 8th ed. London: Bailiere Tindall Books; 1981.

6. Binder SA. Applications of low- and high-voltage electrotherapeutic currents. In: Wolf SL: *Electrotherapy*. Edinburg, Scotland: Churchill Livingstone; 1981.

7. Kloth LC, Cummings JP. *Electrotherapeutic Terminology in Physical Therapy.* Section on Clinical Electrophysiology and the American Physical Therapy Association, Alexandria, VA:1990.

8. Lake DA. Neuromuscular electrical stimulation: an overview and its application in the treatment of sports injuries. *Sports Med*. 1992;13:320.

9. Bowman BR, Baker LL. Effects of waveform parameters on comfort during transcutaneous neuromuscular electrical stimulation. *Ann Biomed Eng*. 1985;13:59.

10. Baker LL, et al. Effect of carrier frequency on comfort with medium frequency electrical stimulation (abstract). *Phys Ther*. 1979;69:373.

11. Karselis T. *Descriptive Medical Electronics and Instrumentation*. Thorofare, NJ: SLACK Incorporated. 1973:12.

12. Alon G, De Domenico F. *High Voltage Stimulation: An Integrated Approach to Clinical Electrotherapy*. Chattanooga, TN: Chattanooga Corporation, 1987.

13. Forster A, Palastange N. *Clayton's Electrotherapy: Theory and Practice.* 8th ed. London: Bailliere Tindall Books; 1981.

14. Wadsworth J, Chanmugam A. *Electrophysical Agents in Physiotherapy: Therapeutic and Diagnostic Use.* 2nd ed. Marrickville: Science Press; 1983.

15. Mehreteab TA. Therapeutic electricity. In: Hecox B. *Physical Agents, A Comprehensive Text for Physical Therapists*. Norwalk, CT: Appleton & Lange; 1994; 225-283.

16. Gracanin F, Trnkoxzy A. Optimal stimulation parameters for minimum pain in the chronic stimulation of innervated muscle. *Arch Phys Med Rehabil*. 1975;56:243.

17. Alon G, De Domenico G. *High Voltage Stimulation: An Integrated Approach to clinical electrotherapy*. Chattanooga, TN: Chattanooga Corporation, 1987.

18. DeVahl J. Neuromuscular electrical stimulation (NMES) in rehabilitation. In: Gersh MR ed. *Electrotherapy in Rehabilitation*. Philadelphia, PA: FA Davis: 1992:218-268.

19. Charman RA. Cellular reception and emission of electromagnetic signals. *Physiotherapy* 76:509,1990.

20. Benton LA. *Functional Electrical Stimulation: A Practical Clinical Guide.* 2nd ed. Ranchos Los Amigos Rehabilitation Engineering Center, Downey, CA; 1981.

21. Leo K. Perceived comfort levels of modulated versus conventional TENS current. *Phys Ther.* (abstr). 1984;64:745.

22. Halstead LS, Seager SW, Houston JM, Whitesell K, Dennis M, Nance PW. Relief of spasticity in SCI men and women using rectal probe electrostimulation. *Paraplegia.* 1993;31(11):715-721.

23. Karnes JL, Mendel FC, Fish DR. Effects of low voltage pulsed current on edema formationin frog hind limbs following impact injury. *Phys Ther.* 1992;72:273.

24. De Domenico G. *Interferential Stimulation (monograph).* Chattanooga,TN: Chattanooga Group; 1988.

25. McCulloch JM, Kloth LC, Feedar JA eds. *Wound Healing: Alternatives in Management.* 2nd ed. Philadelphia, PA: FA Davis; 1995:84.

26. Myklebust B, Robinson AF. Instrumentation. In: Snyder-Mackler L, Robinson AJ eds. *Clinical Electrophysiology, Electrotherapy and Electrophysiologic Testing.* Baltimore, MD: Williams & Wilkins; 1989:31-32, 40-41.

27. Baker LL, Bowman BR, McNeal DR. Effects of wave form on comfort during neuromuscular stimulation. *Clin Orthop.* 1988;223:75.

28. Binder SA. Applications of low-and high-voltage electrotherapeutic currents. In: Wolf SL. *Electrotherapy.* Edinburgh, Scotland.: Churchill Livingston;1981.

29. Bowman BR, Baker LL. Effects of waveform parameters on comfort during transcutaneousneruo-muscular electrical stimulation. *Ann Biomed Eng.* 1985;13:59.

30. Benton LA. *Functional Electrical Stimulation: A Practical clinical Guid.* 2nd ed. Ranchos Los Amigos Rehabilitaiton Engineering Center: Downey, CA; 1981.

31. Baker LL, Bowman BR, McNeal DR. Effects of wave form on comfort during neuromuscular stimulation. *Clin Orthop.* 1988;223:75.

32. Davis HL. Is electrostimulation beneficial to denervated muscle? A review of results from basic research. *Physiother Can.* 1983;35:306.

33. Lake DA. Neuromuscular electrical stimulation: An overview and its application in the treatment of sports injuries. *Sports Med.* 1992;13:320.

34. Delitto A, Snyder-Mackler L. Two theories of muscle strength augmentation using percutaneous neuromuscular electrical stimulation. *Ann Biomed Eng.* 1985;13:59.

35. Currier DP, Mann R. Muscular strength development by electrical stimulation in healthy individuals. *Phys Ther.* 1987;63:346.

36. Robinson AJ, Snyder-Mackler L eds. *Clinical Electrophysiology, Electrotherapy and Electrophysiologic Testing,* 2nd ed. Baltimore, MD: Williams & Wilkins; 1995:129-130.

37. Delitto A, Mc Kowan JM, Mc Carthy JA, Shively RA, Rose SJ. Electrically elicited co-contraction of thigh musculature after anterior cruciate ligament surgery. *Phys Ther.* 1988;68(1):45-50.

38. Selkowitz DM. Improvement in isometric strength of the quadriceps femoris muscle after training with electrical stimulation. *Phys Ther.* 1985;6:186.

39. Carley PJ, Wainapel SF. Electrotherapy for acceleration of wound healing: Low-intensity direct current. *Arch Phys Med Rehabil.* 1985;66:443.

40. Feedar JA, Kloth LC, Gentzkow GD. Chronic dermal ulcer healing enhanced with monophasic pulsed electrical stimulation. *Phys Ther.* 1991;71:639.

41. Kloth LC. Physical Modalities in wound management: UVC, therapeutic heating and electrical stimulation. *Ostomy Wound Management.* 1995;41:18.

42. Bettany JA, Fish DR, Mendel FC. Influence of high voltage pulsed direct current on edema formation following impact injury. *Phys Ther.* 1990;70(4):219-224.

43. Mendel FC, Fish DR. New perspectives in edema control via electrical stimulation. *Journal of Athletic Training.* 1993;28:1.

44. Trimble MH, Enoka RM. Mechanisms underlying the training effects associated with neuromuscular electrical stimulation. *Phys Ther.* 1991;71:273.

45. Draper U, Ballard L. Electrical stimulation versus electromyographic biofeedback in the recovery of quadriceps femoris muscle function following anterior cruciate ligament surgery. *Phys Ther.* 1991;71:455.

46. Bettany JA, Newsome L, Stralka S. High voltage pulsed current-effect on edema formation after hyper-flexion injury. *Arch Phys Med Rehabil.* 1993;71:677.

47. Fitzgerald GK, Newsome D. Treatment of a large infected thoracic spine wound using high voltage pulsed monophasic current. *Phys Ther.* 1993;73:355.

48. Gordon TM, Mao J. Muscle atrophy and procedures for training after spinal cord injury. *Phys Ther.* 1994;74:50.

49. Nash HL, Rogers CC. Does electricity speed the healing of non-union fractures. *Physician and Sports Medicine.* 1988;16:156.

50. Stanish WD. The use of electricity in ligament and tendon repair. *Physician and Sports Medicine.* 1985;13:110.

51. Balogun JA. High voltage electrical stimulation in the augmentation of muscle strength: Effects of pulse frequency. *Arch Phys Med Rehabil.* 1993;74:910.

52. Taylor K, Fish DR, Mendel FC, Burton HW. Effect of a single 30-minute treatment of high voltage pulsed current on edema formation in frog hind limbs. *Phys Ther.* 1992;72(1):63-68.

Chapter Ten

Neuromuscular Electrical Stimulation: Applications & Indications

Alfred G. Bracciano, EdD, OTR
David Czupinski, OTR, CHT

Learning Objectives

1. Describe the clinical application of electrical stimulation in rehabilitation.
2. Outline and discuss the clinical reasoning process used to determine selection of NMES and appropriate parameters.
3. Discuss the issues and factors which impact on NMES efficacy.
4. Discuss the indications and contraindications for NMES use.
5. Identify appropriate electrode placement for treatment protocols.

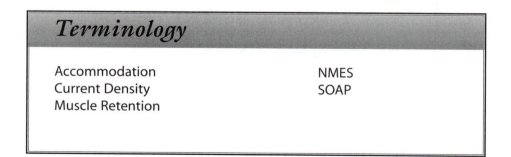

Terminology

Accommodation	NMES
Current Density	SOAP
Muscle Retention	

Background

Clinically, neuromuscular electrical stimulation (NMES) is used to selectively evoke muscle contraction through stimulation of the intact or partially intact peripheral nervous system. NMES can be used to strengthen or prevent disuse atrophy during immobilization or inactivity, maintain or improve range of motion, facilitate voluntary motor control, decrease spasticity and muscle spasm, and as a substitute for orthosis.

Stimulating to Maintain Muscle Mass

Research over the years has shown that the electrical stimulation of healthy, innervated tissue showed little difference from muscle tissue put through traditional exercise and maximum isometric contraction. However, when faced with a patient demonstrating submaximal effort, such as a patient who is holding back due to anticipated pain, electrical stimulation may be a viable intervention until maximum effort can be achieved through traditional activity and exercise. Strength gains occur through the overload principle.[1] Overload occurs during exercise programs consisting of a small number of high intensity contractions, for example, a minimum of 70% of a maximal contraction x10 repetitions. Patients with orthopedic and traumatic injuries appear to demonstrate greater strength gains with NMES than with straight exercise alone. Combining NMES with occupational activity can further enhance gains. Electrical stimulation should not replace voluntary muscle contraction but is most effective when used as an adjunct to exercise and activity.[2,3]

Stimulation to Maintain or Gain ROM

Electrical stimulation may be employed on patients who demonstrate moderate to high levels of spasticity. This may occur more frequently with neurologically impaired clients or with orthopedic patients. In neurologically impaired populations increased spasticity may result in decreasing ROM to joints affecting their occupational performance. Patients with mild levels of spasticity may respond to passive range of motion activities better than moderate or severe spasticity. Traditional ROM techniques in home exercise programs, particularly when spasticity is moderate or severe, may become ineffective. NMES can be used as an adjunct to passive range of motion and in conjunction with serial casting or splinting. NMES can be applied to either the spastic muscle or the antagonist. With appropriate parameters, this results in a muscle contraction sufficient to take the joint through its complete range of motion. In applying electrical stimulation to an individual with severe spasticity, care should be taken to use a long "ramp up" time. Lengthening the ramp up time will decrease the likelihood of stimulating the spastic response and will result in a more balanced muscle contraction. As with all uses of electrical stimulation the practitioner should be fully versed in the treatment protocol necessary with clear goals outlined.

Electrical Stimulation to Facilitate Voluntary Motor Control

There have been several studies evaluating the effectiveness of electrical stimulation in the treatment of healthy individuals, and with orthopedically or neurologically involved patients. Several studies have shown the improvement of functional performance following electrical stimulation. NMES can facilitate improvement of performance and efficiency of muscle recruitment.[4-6] Electrical stimulation as a muscle facilitation technique works best when it is part of a highly structured program with active patient participation. It has been postulated that one reason for its effectiveness may be due to the increase in sensory information to the central nervous system. This increased sensory feedback may result in the individual's increased ability to activate specific muscle groups.[7-9] A voluntary contraction which is enhanced and augmented by NMES can be used to facilitate and strengthen a weak response.[10-13] Incorporation of the NMES and stimulation at the appropriate time within an occupational task strengthens the results and outcomes. Utilizing NMES during functional activity such as grasp and release, or for upper extremity positioning to recruit weak muscle groups, will be rewarding to the patient and reinforce the reeducation of the motor pattern.

Electrical Stimulation for the Management of Spasticity

Research into the use of electrical stimulation for the control of spasticity has demonstrated only short term control in neurologically impaired patients due to the underlying CNS abnormality. Long-term control is usually not achieved through the use of NMES. NMES treatment protocols for spasticity interrupt the abnormal cycle that stimulates the motor neuron through muscle fatigue using a high-frequency stimulation. ROM may improve due to a break in the pain-spasm cycle of spasticity. Numerous studies performed on both agonist and antagonist spastic muscles indicate that stimulation of the antagonist muscles causes an inhibition of the agonist. Even with stimulation of the agonist, however, minimal long-term improvement is demonstrated due to the underlying pathology.[14-19]

Electrical Stimulation Used as an Orthotic

Electrical stimulation has been used effectively in place of orthotics and in conjunction with bracing to increase patient motor control and to facilitate occupational performance. Because the use of electrical stimulation is to gain control of function of targeted muscle groups, it is often referred to as functional electrical stimulation (FES). Electrical stimulation can be an effective substitute for orthotics when activating innervated but paretic, or paralyzed muscles. FES has been used to facilitate standing and ambulation in spinal cord injured patients, for idiopathic scoliosis, and as a dorsiflexion assist with patients with CVA.[20-22] An intervention often used clinically, incorporates electrical stimulation as a substitute for orthotics in the treatment of CVA. Training weakened or paretic musculature in a hemiplegic shoulder may reduce shoulder subluxation.

Factors Affecting Neuromuscular Electrical Stimulation

There is a wide variety of electrical equipment available for clinical use. Clinicians should be familiar with the type and parameters of the equipment available in their department before using electrical stimulation as part of their overall treatment program. It is vital to remember that use of electrical stimulation does not take precedence over engagement of the patient in appropriate activities and occupations but is most effective when used in conjunction with occupation. Clinicians should be familiar with the operation of the equipment available to them and thoroughly review the operating manual.

There are some basic considerations which need to be taken into account prior to using neuromuscular stimulation as part of the treatment protocol. The amplitude, pulse duration, resistance/impedance, electrode size and placement, and the frequency will all affect the quantity or the amount of current required to stimulate motor nerves causing depolarization. The frequency and duty cycle affect the quality of the muscle contraction, the strength of the contraction and the rate of fatigue. The amplitude will provide the subjective comfort level and determine the magnitude of the sensory or motor response. The pulse duration will also affect the subjective comfort level of the stimulation and will also affect the current density and release of endorphins. The longer the pulse duration, the greater the penetration and release of endorphins. Rise times which are set for a gradual onset facilitate patient comfort by avoiding a sudden onset of the stimulation. [23-25] Longer rise times between 6-8 seconds should be used with more spastic muscles.

The duty cycle (on/off time) should be adjusted based on the condition of the patient. Historically, a 1:5 ratio is recommended for strengthening but a 1:3 ratio may be used for a debilitated patient; a 1:2 ratio for an individual with average musculature; and a 1:1 ratio for athletic or conditioned individuals; a 1:1 ratio can also be used to fatigue muscles. The longer the on time, the greater the exercise that occurs. An objective method of documenting improvement in a patient is through documenting a decrease in the on/off time. Other primary factors include:

1. *Current Density:* The amount passing into the skin from an electrode is affected by the size of the electrode. The smaller the electrode the higher the current density per square inch. When the same amount of current is used, the larger the electrode the lower the current is per square inch.

2. *Accommodation:* This is the automatic rise in the threshold of excitation resulting from a gradually increasing stimulus applied to excitable tissue. As the tissue is stimulated it will accommodate to the stimulus, resulting in more stimulus being necessary to achieve the desired result or a decreased response to the same amount of stimulus.

3. *Electrode Placement:* In stimulating healthy innervated muscle tissue one can use either monopolar or bipolar techniques. Monopolar stimulation uses a small active electrode over the motor point of the muscle. A dispersive pad is used on the same side of the body. The dispersive pad is usually larger to decrease the current density. This allows a higher current density under the active electrode, thus stimulating the motor point with greater comfort. Bipolar stimulation utilizes two electrodes of approximately the same size. They are placed over a single muscle group or group of muscles at each end of the muscle belly. The current is then passed through the muscle belly and results in contraction of the muscle.

4. *Skin Tolerance:* Skin tolerance to electric stimulation is limited. If the current is too high under the electrode a burn may result. Proper electrode preparation is necessary to achieve even stimulus. If the electrode is not properly prepared uneven current flow could result. Improper electrode preparation and placement may result in higher current density in some areas and a burn may occur.

5. *Tolerance of Muscle Tissue to Electric Stimulation:* Following repeated stimulation to achieve muscle contraction, fatigue of the muscle will result. This is usually

noted by tremors in the muscle during contraction and a decrease in strength. To continue stimulation it may be necessary to increase the intensity to achieve a contraction. Continually increasing the intensity during a treatment session would result in little benefit and possible damage to the muscles.

Contraindications for NMES

There are minimal contraindications for the use of electrical stimulation. When using NMES it should be noted that there are some specific conditions for which stimulation is contraindicated or have precautions against the use of stimulation. Precautions and contraindications should always be a consideration during the evaluation when goals, objectives, and treatment interventions are being considered. Contraindications and precautions for the use of electrical stimulation include:

1. Over the thoracic region as it may interfere with heart activity
2. Patients with pacemakers
3. In areas of phrenic nerve or bladder stimulators
4. Over the carotid sinus as this may cause cardiac arrhythmias
5. With hypertensive or hypotensive patients
6. Peripheral vascular disorders such as venous thrombosis or thrombophlebitis
7. Patients with cancer, infection, tuberculosis, or active hemorrhage
8. Pregnant women
9. Near diathermy devices
10. Obese patients with excessive adipose tissue
11. Patients unable to provide clear feedback regarding the level of stimulation such as infants, senile patients, or individuals with mental disorders
12. Over areas with pathology of the cell body, ie, polio
13. Over areas with pathology of the myelin sheath ie, diabetic neuropathy, MS, peripheral neuropathy.
14. Over areas with pathology of the synapse points between muscle and nerve, ie, myasthenia gravis
15. Over areas with pathology within the muscle, ie, muscular dystrophy
16. Caution should be used in areas of absent or diminished sensation
17. Patients with skin conditions such as eczema, psoriasis, acne, dermatitis
18. Over or near superficial metal pins, plates, or hardware [26,27]

NMES Applications

There are a wide variety of applications for NMES (Figures 10-1 to 10-3). The therapist should complete a thorough evaluation of the patient to determine objective measurements and function to assist in identifying appropriate goals and interventions. NMES is most effective when there is an intact or partially intact peripheral nerve pathway. Therapists should be aware of the contraindications and precautions of electrical stimulation and should be well acquainted with the equipment that is available to them in their clinic. As there is a wide range of equipment available, the therapist should be familiar with the particular features of the selected equipment and thoroughly

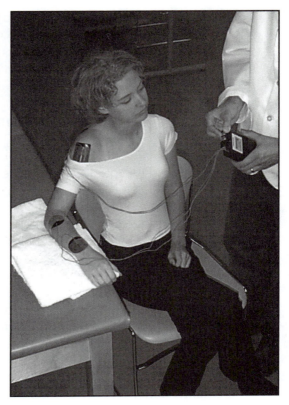

Figure 10-1. Neuromuscular electrical stimulation using a two channel, four electrode configuration. Electrode placements would be used for treating shoulder subluxation and for facilitating wrist extension. Adequate amount of electrode gel is necessary for patient comfort. Amplitude is increased to provide a muscle contraction.

review the equipment manual. Informing the patient and family as to the goals and objectives as well as the possible subjective feelings which the patient may experience when applying electrical stimulation will help to allay the patient's fears.

Though there are a number of potential applications for NMES, we will discuss those most frequently used by occupational therapists. It should be noted that there are a variety of applications and possible protocols for specific muscle groups, and the clinician is encouraged to explore other treatment options.

The following protocols are formulated to provide recommended settings for wave form, intensity, pulse duration, frequency, on/off time, treatment time and possible functional activities. These settings may vary with patients, and are intended to guide the therapist's clinical reasoning.

Maintaining or Increasing Active Range of Motion in Patients with Hemiplegia

Maintaining or increasing active range of motion in patients who have experienced a stroke can be accomplished using either asymmetrical or symmetrical biphasic waveforms. Therapists should have a good understanding of the anatomy of muscles and their innervations in order to stimulate the muscles effectively. Stimulation of the muscle provides a method of actively exercising the muscle in those patients unable to voluntarily contract the muscle.

Stimulation of the muscle in patients with hemiplegia prevents or can reverse atrophy which occurs due to disuse or immobility, and facilitate peripheral circulation preventing fibrosis. Additionally, the stimulation provides the patient with proprioceptive

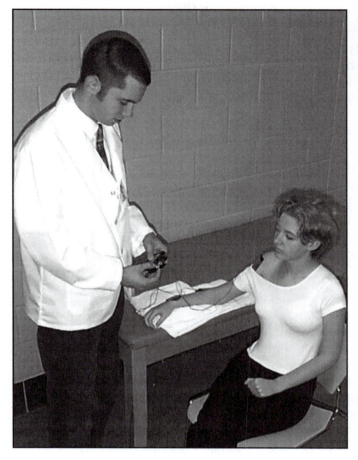

Figure 10-2. Neuromuscular electrical stimulation. Amplitude, pulse duration, resistance/impedance, electrode size and placement, and frequency affect the amount of current needed to stimulate motor nerves causing depolorization.

and visual feedback which can be motivating to those patients with limited movement. Use of electrical stimulation for shoulder subluxation or flaccid paralysis following a CVA assists in maintaining approximation of the humoral head in the glenohumoral joint.

The therapist should select the muscle or muscle group to be stimulated. Pulse duration is usually set at 200-300 microseconds, with the frequency between 25 and 35 pulses per second. Frequencies should be chosen which achieve the desired outcome, yet are comfortable to the patient. The intensity is increased to achieve tetany, which allows for a fair + muscle grade in the desired muscle. The on/off ratio should be 1:3 or higher to allow muscles a chance to recover between contractions. Treatment time is usually 30 minutes BID to TID for 5 sessions per week. Treatment should continue for 3-4 weeks with re-evaluation occurring to determine treatment effectiveness.

To facilitate effectiveness of the intervention and carry-over, neuromuscular stimulators may often be used as part of a home exercise program. Proper patient and family training is a necessity to ensure that the patient and care-giver are familiar and comfortable with electrode placement, skin care, and the stimulating parameters of the equipment. Specific pad placement for muscle groups will be discussed later.

Facilitation of Tendon Excursion

Orthopedic or neurological conditions which limit tendon excursion can be approached using either asymmetrical or symmetrical biphasic pulse waveforms.

A thorough understanding of the patient's condition, particularly if surgical intervention has occurred, and the stage of wound healing is of vital importance. Again, a complete evaluation and review of the patient's history is required to assist in correctly identifying appropriate goals and interventions. To facilitate tendon excursion for innervated muscles, the pulse duration is set between 200-300 microseconds, with a frequency of 25-50 pulses per second. Intensity is increased to achieve maximal contraction of the muscle so that a comfortable tendon excursion is noted. Intensity should never be set above the tolerable level of the patient. Lower intensity levels can be used at the start of treatment and increased as tolerance improves. On/off duration should be a 1:3 ratio. The recommended treatment time is for 30 minute sessions 2-3 times daily, over a period of 3-5 days per week. Electrical stimulation may not be indicated once the patient can achieve a maximal contraction of the target muscle voluntarily, and reevaluation of treatment goals and interventions should occur.

Facilitation or Reeducation of Voluntary Muscle Function

Use of electrical stimulation for muscle reeducation may be effective following neurologic injury, and orthopedic surgery such as tendon transfers. The therapist should determine if the patient displays limitation of movement due to immobilization or disuse atrophy, weakness, or due to pain. Stimulation can be used to facilitate weak movement or to provide stability to a targeted muscle group. The therapist should identify the target muscle or muscle group. The waveform can be either asymmetrical or symmetrical biphasic pulse. The pulse duration is set between 200-300 microseconds, with a frequency between 25-50 pulses per second. The on/off ratio should be 1:3 dependent on identified goals. The intensity should be increased to achieve a tetanic contraction of appropriate size.

As always, electrode placement is of great importance, and the stimulator should be turned off and the electrodes relocated if the contraction is incorrect or the selected muscle group is not responding. During stimulation, the patient should attempt to actively move the targeted muscle group in conjunction with the stimulation. As greater voluntary control develops, the intensity can be gradually reduced to a sensory level and the patient instructed to actively contract the muscle with each "on" cycle. Treatment sessions are usually 30 minutes, 1-2 times per day, and can extend over 3-5 days per week.

NMES for Relaxation of Muscle Spasm

As discussed earlier, NMES can be used to decrease the pain and tension accompanied by muscle spasm or spasticity. Effectiveness of this technique with the neurologically involved patient is usually of short benefit due to the underlying pathology. NMES can, however, be used with success in those orthopedic patients who are having muscle spasm due to injury. NMES is typically used to fatigue a muscle thus relaxing the spasm. Its most notable use is in the muscles of the shoulder which may be limiting functional movement due to pain and spasm. The wave form can be either asymmetrical or symmetrical biphasic pulse. The pulse duration is 300 microseconds with a frequency between 30-60 pulses per second. The intensity is increased to patient tolerance and to achieve a gentle contraction. To achieve fatigue of the muscle group, the on/off ratio should be 1:1. The electrodes should be placed over the motor point with stimulation continuing until muscle fatigue is noted.

NMES for Inhibition of Spasticity

Inhibition of spasticity is dependent on the underlying pathology and degree of spasticity in the patient. Though a relaxation can occur in the neurologically involved individual, the underlying cause of the spasticity may limit the overall effectiveness of the intervention. A thorough evaluation of the patient and the underlying cause should be completed to identify those areas which may respond better to the stimulation and have a prolonged effect. Spasticity is associated with hypertonia, hyperactive deep tendon reflexes and clonus, and is difficult to manage.

NMES for decreasing spasticity in the neurologically involved patient can be used as an adjunct method to cooling, vibration, and serial casting or splinting. Reductions in muscle tone following stimulation can last for a minimum of 30 minutes to a maximum of 6 hours. There are three primary methods of approaching the problem.

1. *Stimulation of the antagonist muscle to the spastic muscle.* The treatment proto col is the same as described in increasing ROM. Stimulation is carried out three times daily for 30 minutes with expected results of 10 minutes to 2 hours of relief from spasticity.
2. *Stimulation of the spastic muscle directly in order to achieve an overall muscle fatigue.* This protocol is the same as stimulating the antagonist only stimulation is to the spastic muscle directly.
3. *Stimulating the antagonist and spastic muscle alternately.* This protocol is the same as that used to increase AROM. The stimulator is set to alternately stimulate agonist and antagonist muscles. An additional application which may prove to be effective is stimulation of the acupuncture points, though the neurophysiological basis for its effectiveness is not clearly understood.

NMES to Improve Strengthening or Prevent Atrophy from Disuse

As previously stated, NMES may be used when reinnervation has occurred and the patient is unable to achieve voluntary contraction without electric stimulation. The waveform can be asymmetrical or symmetrical biphasic. The pulse duration is 300 microseconds with a frequency between 25-35 pulses per second. The intensity should be gradually increased to the maximum tolerated contraction with an on/off time of 1:1 or 1:2. The recommended treatment is 10-20 repetitive contractions, 3-5 times per week. Treatment is usually continued until the patient can achieve maximal contraction of the target muscle without electric stimulation.

NMES for Use in Treatment of Joint Contracture

Joint contractures also present a challenging problem for the clinician. A complete evaluation to determine the cause of the contracture as well as the total active or passive movement available is necessary to aid in determining the appropriate approach. The end-feel is also of importance as a bony block or hard end-feel may limit a positive outcome. As always, a thorough review of the patient's history, surgical intervention and underlying pathology will help guide treatment goals.

The treatment protocol used in treating a joint contracture is essentially the same protocol utilized for increasing AROM. Stimulation parameters are essentially the same with the addition of serial casting which can be modified with openings over the electrode sites. Serial casting can be reapplied in greater degrees of motion as progress is made.

NMES in the Treatment of the Hemiplegic Shoulder

Electrical stimulation is an effective intervention and is used to increase or maintain tone in the affected shoulder following a CVA. The electrical stimulator acts as a substitute to the traditional arm sling which many patients wear due to shoulder subluxation and flaccid paralysis of the affected extremity. Stimulation of the deltoid reapproximates the humoral head in the glenohumoral joint decreasing subluxation of the shoulder.

Treatment parameters are the same as those used for muscle strengthening and facilitation. Bipolar electrode placement is over the supraspinatus and posterior deltoid muscles. A quadripolar pattern can also be used with electrode placement on the motor points of the deltoid and the three rotator cuff muscles, the supraspinatus, infraspinatus and teres minor. The on/off ratio for a power program is .1 to 1 second for a power program, or 1.5 to 5 seconds for a strengthening program. NMES is effective in reducing shoulder subluxation, but is less effective in decreasing shoulder pain associated with the hemiplegic shoulder.

Electrode Placement

Electrode placement for NMES will vary depending on what muscle group is being stimulated and the goal of the program. A thorough understanding of the kinesiology, muscle insertion and innervation of the targeted muscle as well as the underlying pathology is necessary to ensure appropriate response of the tissue. There is a wide variety of potential applications and electrode placements for NMES dependent upon the identified goals and objectives.

The following electrode placements provide a sampling of the possible electrode placements for use with NMES and is intended to serve as a general guide for some of the more common programs used in occupational therapy.

Electrode Placements and General Parameters

- 1-12 are located on the posterior arm and are used in stimulating extensor muscles (Figure 10-3).
- A-H are located on the anterior side and are used in stimulating the flexor muscle groups (Figure 10-4).

1. Over the supraspinatus muscle
2. Over the triceps muscle belly
3. Over the long head of the triceps muscles
4. Over the triceps tendon at the musculotendonis junction
5. Between the motor points of the ECU, ECRB and ECRL muscles
6. Over the lateral epicondyle
7. Motor point of the ECRL
8. Between motor points of EDC and EIP muscles
9. Radial dorsal wrist
10. Dorsal wrist
11. Ulnar dorsal wrist
12. Motor points of posterior interossei muscles

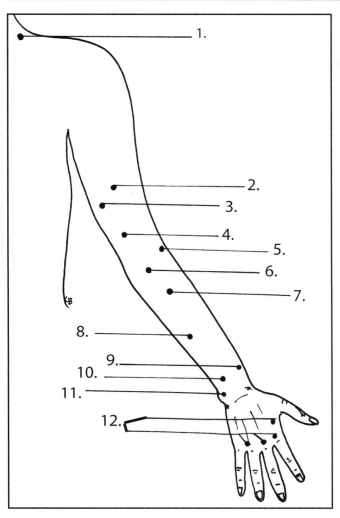

Figure 10-3. Neuromuscular electrical stimulation electrode placements— posterior view for stimulation of upper extremity extensor muscles. Illustration by Kim Bartlett. Used with permission.

A. Between motor points of FCR and FCU
B. Motor point of brachioradialis
C. Between motor points of FDS and FDP
D. Motor point of FPL
E. Radial volar wrist
F. Volar wrist
G. Ulnar volar wrist
H. Ulnar nerve at Guyons Canal
I. Motor point of FPB

NMES Treatment Guide

The following protocols are recommended guidelines for the use of NMES. For ease and clarity of application, the electrodes are labeled positive and negative. Because the protocols are using a biphasic waveform, the pulse is bidirectional. Either the negative or positive electrode could be placed on either motor point of the protocols. Some electrode leads use the colors of black and red, or brown and white. The clinician should

Figure 10-4. Neuromuscular electrical stimulation electrode placement for stimulation of upper extremity flexor muscle groups. Illustration by Kim Bartlett. Used with permission.

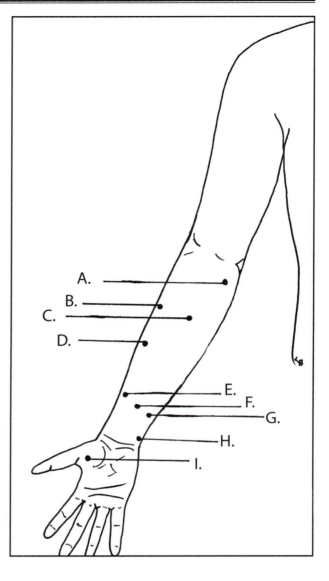

review the manufacturer's information on the equipment being used and apply the guidelines based on their equipment (Table 10-1).

Incorporating Functional Activities with Electrical Stimulation

As with any physical agent, neuromuscular electrical stimulation is most effectively used as an adjunct to the occupational therapy plan. NMES will be more effective when combined with voluntary movement facilitating an individual's occupational performance. NMES has an extrinsic value to the treatment process but incorporating active, functional activities and interventions adds intrinsic value and motivation to the treatment protocol for the patient. Many of the uses of neuromuscular electrical stimulation in occupational therapy are based on using the stimulation for functional electrical stimulation and activities. NMES can be used to facilitate movement and muscular contractions in patients with minimal activity, as well as being used to strengthen or

Table 10-1. Recommended Electrode Placements for NMES of the Upper Extremity.

Treatment Protocol	Wave form	- Pad Location (motor point=mp)	+ Pad Location (dispersive)
Wrist flexion	asymmetrical biphasic	small electrode over (A) mp of FCR, FCU	(F) volar aspect of the wrist
Power grasp	symmetrical biphasic	small active electrode over (C) mp between FCS and FDP	(H) ulnar nerve
Thumb IP flexion	asymmetrical biphasic	small electrode over (D) mp of the FPL	Larger inactive electrode over (F) volar wrist
Composite Thumb Flexion	symmetrical biphasic	small electrode over (D) motor point of FPL	(F) volar wrist
Lumbricals 3 & 4	asymmetrical biphasic	small electrode over (C) motor point btw FDS &FDP	inactive electrode over (F) volar wrist
Combination with Power Grasp and Extrinsic Flexion w/ w. Lumbrical 3 & 4	asymmetrical biphasic	small active electrode over (C) btw. motor points of FDS &FDP, and (H) ulnar nerve	dispersive electrode over (E) and (G) ulnar & radial aspect of volar wrist
Wrist extension	asymmetrical biphasic	small electrode (5) btw motor points of ECRL, ECRB, and ECU	large electrode at (1) dorsal wrist
Wrist extension with associated EDC facilitation	asymmetrical biphasic	small electrode over (5) motor point btw. ECRB, ECRL & ECU muscles	large electrode over (6) lateral epicondyle
Digital extension	asymmetrical biphasic wave form	small electrode over (8) motor point btw. EDC & EIP	large electrode over (10) dorsal wrist
Elbow extension	symmetrical biphasic	small electrode over (3) motor point of the medial head of of the triceps	same size electrode over (4) between the motor points of the long head and lateral head of the triceps

Table 10-1, Continued			
Treatment Protocol	**Waveform**	**- Pad Location (motor point =mp)**	**+ Pad Location (dispersive)**
1st dorsal interossei	asymmetrical biphasic	small electrode place place at (12) the 1st intrinsic muscle; placement can be modified for 2nd, 3rd, 4th, interossi by moving the smaller electrode over appropriate muscle	large electrode at (10) dorsal wrist
Composite digital and wrist extension	symmetrical biphasic	small electrode over (7) motor point btw ECRL, ECRB & ECU	electrode placed at (8) btw motor points of EDC & EIP
Wrist extension with grasp (two channels & four leads) [use alternating channel	asymmetrical biphasic	Pad placement for wrist extensors and extrinsic digital flexors	Pad placement for wrist extensors and extrinsic digital flexors

augment weak voluntary movement. Used functionally, NMES can be incorporated to strengthen a particular motor response, such as grasp and release activities of the finger flexors and extensors. NMES is also frequently used as a substitute for shoulder slings, with electrode placement being used to strengthen shoulder flexion and abduction. Treatment protocols for the shoulder may also provide some measure of pain relief to those patients with shoulder/hand syndrome. Patients who display essentially flaccid musculature of the shoulder due to hemiplegia may benefit from stimulation to the posterior deltoid and supraspinatus muscle to increase tone and decrease subluxation. With any of the upper extremity protocols for strengthening or facilitation, incorporating a hand switch to trigger the stimulation can be an effective method for table activities, and for producing functional grasp and release activities. Using bifurcated leads, the therapist can effectively target up to four muscle groups, facilitating a wide range of motion and activities. Creativity and analysis of the movement patterns desired are a necessary component of the evaluation and formative assessment.

As the spectrum of conditions and applications for NMES use in the treatment process will vary, the occupational therapist must be creative and adept at analyzing the activity and movement which is being facilitated by the stimulation to determine appropriate interventions. Though the activity and technique may be different for each client, the underlying benefit of greater effectiveness of NMES when combined with functional, active movement will be consistent with nearly all interventions and applications. Patient compliance and engagement in the treatment process and in setting appropriate and achievable goals is vital to success.

Documentation

As with any other intervention, clear and concise documentation is important to ensure that there is a complete chronological record of the client's condition and course of intervention. Appropriate documentation aids in facilitating communication with other team members and provides an objective means of determining the appropriateness and effectiveness of the intervention.

Documentation can include a narrative format or more commonly, a SOAP (S=subjective; O=objective; A=assessment; P=plan) format. When documenting the treatment parameters for NMES, the subjective information which is documented should include any subjective information or comments related to the therapist by the patient. Objectively, the therapist should document the target area being treated and the location of the electrodes; the overall treatment time for the stimulation; the treatment goal or goals with the identified electrode placement; and all of the treatment parameters including: the type of the device used, the on/off time, ramp on/off and time, and the intensity. Specific treatment results or characteristics of the stimulation should also be identified and documented: volitional contraction, static resistance, or during an activity.

As with any therapeutic intervention, the documentation should present an external reader with a clear and concise record of what was done and how the patient responded to the intervention. Making sure that the documentation clearly demonstrates the relationship between the use of NMES and occupational performance areas will also assist in identifying the need and appropriateness of the intervention to external auditors such as third party payers.

Summary

NMES can be an effective adjunct in the treatment of a variety of conditions. NMES can facilitate muscle contraction, improve or enhance the development of strength, reeducate muscles, and assist in the training of new muscle function. With less muscle atrophy, the patient displays better ability to voluntarily contract their muscles leading to better clinical function, facilitating occupational performance.

Indirect benefits of NMES include increased blood flow, improved venous and lymphatic drainage and prevention of/or loosening adhesion formation. NMES can be effective in decreasing disuse atrophy, increasing ROM, facilitating functional use of muscles, decreasing tone in spastic musculature and facilitating muscular contraction.

Through evaluation and assessment, the therapist must identify the need and goal of NMES as part of the overall treatment process. NMES should be incorporated into the occupational therapy intervention with regard to the significance and importance of volitional movement and occupation.

There are a number of electrical stimulators available on the market, and it is the clinician's responsibility to fully evaluate and understand the equipment which will be used with the client. The clinician also must be aware of the indications and contraindications to the use of NMES to safely and effectively incorporate electrical stimulation into treatment. NMES can be a useful technology and adjunct to occupational therapy, enhancing occupational performance, facilitating independence, and improving patient outcomes.

Case Study

Mr.P is a 72 y/o male with a right middle cerebral artery thrombosis 5 weeks prior to his initial evaluation. Mr. P was an active individual before the stroke, continuing to farm, garden, and maintain an active lifestyle such as travelling and involvement with his church. Mr. P is married, his wife is in good health, and he has friends and family who live near him and assist him as needed. Mr. P has had good functional return since the initial onset, he is able to ambulate using a quad cane and AFO. Assessment reveals active movement in the left upper extremity with better control distally. He has weak finger flexion and extension with weak grasp. Movement at the biceps and triceps is nearly full. Mr. P's primary difficulty is the lack of strength and endurance in the left shoulder. He displays approximately 65 degrees of active shoulder flexion and 70 degrees of abduction. He displays a one finger subluxation and has been complaining of pain in the shoulder. A friend told him that he should be wearing a sling to "take the pressure off the shoulder", but he is concerned that his arm will "stiffen" if it is immobilized. He has been working on arm/hand placement activities with moderate success, but decreased endurance in the shoulder has limited his ability.

After further assessment of the shoulder integrity, strength, sensation, skin condition, and obtaining a medical history from the patient and his family, treatment using NMES for functional electrical stimulation of the shoulder was implemented. Therapeutic goals were to decrease the pain in the shoulder, facilitate active shoulder movement, decrease subluxation and possible dependence on a sling. Sling use should be avoided in this type of patient, because posturally, use of a sling will cause internal rotation and adduction of the arm. FES consisted of active electrode placement over the posterior deltoid on the proximal one-third of the arm. The indifferent electrode was cut and placed to fit over the supraspinous fosa, above the scapula and over the supraspinatus. Intensity was increased to achieve tetany and a strengthening protocol was used. The electrical stimulation facilitated a more normal alignment of the humerus with the glenoid fossa, while allowing free functional use and movement of the forearm and hand. As the strength continued to return in the shoulder, electrode placements to stimulate shoulder flexion and abduction were implemented paired with reaching and grasping activities to reinforce the patterns and gains. For shoulder flexion and abduction, both electrodes were placed on the proximal third of the anterior arm, below the acromium. A space of a minimum of 1 inch was maintained between the electrodes, and intensity was increased to achieve a contraction, with a strengthening protocol used. As Mr. P became more independent and functional, he was given a NMES unit for home use and instructed in electrode placement and strengthening protocols. Mr. P was eventually able to actively grasp and reach for objects in a controlled and fluid movement. He gained functional shoulder flexion and abduction to 100 degrees and used the stimulator as needed.

References

1. Delitto A, Snyder-Mackler L. Two theories of muscle strength augmentation using percutaneous electrical stimulation. *Phys Ther*. 1990;70:158.

2. Hobler CK. Case study: Reduction of chronic posttraumatic knee edema using interferential stimulation. *Athletic Training*. 1991;26:364.

3. Selkowitz DM. Improvement in isometric strength of the quadriceps femoris muscle after training with electrical stimulation. *Phys Ther.* 1988;65:186.

4. Bogataj U, Gros N, Malezic M, et al. Restoration of gait during two to three weeks of therapy with multi-channel electrical stimulation. *Phys Ther.* 1989; 69(5):319-327.

5. Crastam B, Larson E, Previc T. Improvement of gait following functional electrical stimulation. *Scan J Rehabil Med.* 1977;9:7-13.

6. Parker K, Baumgarten J. Upper extremity control in Rancho Los Amigos rehab engineering, Downey, Ca: *Annual Report of Progress.* 1981;4.

7. Winchester P, Montgomery J. Effect of feedback stimulation training and cyclical electrical stimulation on knee extension in hemiplegic patients. *Phys Ther.* 1983;63:1096-1103.

8. Bowman B, Baker L, Waters R. Positional feedback and electrical stimulation: an automated treatment for the hemiplegic wrist. *Arch Phys Med Rehabil.* 1979;60:497-502.

9. Baker LL, Yeh C. Electrical stimulation of wrist and fingers for hemiplegic patients. *Phys Ther.* 1979;59:1495-1499.

10. Baker LL, Parker K, Sanderson D. Neuromuscular electrical stimulation for the head-injured patient. *Phys Ther.* 1983;63:1967,

11. Craik Rl, Cozzens B, Miyazaki S. Enhancement of swing phase clearance through sensory stimulation. *Ann Conf Rehabil Eng.* 1981;4:217.

12. Malezic M, Stanic U, Kljajic M. Multichannel electrical stimulation of gait in motor disabled patients. *Orthopedics*:1984;1187.

13. Bajd T, Kralj A, Turk R. Standing-up for a healthy subject and a paraplegic patient. *J Biomechanics.* 1982;15:1.

14. Cranstam B, Larsson LE. Electrical stimulation in patients with spasticity. *Electroencephalogr Clin Neurophysiol Soc Proc.* 1975;38:214.

15. Dimitrijevic MR, Nathan PW. Studies of spasticity in man. 4. Changes in flexion reflex with repetitive cutaneous stimulation in spinal man. *Brain.* 1970;93(4):743-768.

16. Levine MG, Knott M, Kabat H. Relaxation of spasticity by electrical stimulation of antagonist muscles. *Arch Phys Med.* 1952;33:668.

17. Fulbright JS. Electrical stimulation to reduce chronic toe-flexor hypertonicity. A case report. *Phys Ther.* 1984;64:523.

18. Lee WJ, McGovern JP, Duval EN. Continuous tetanizing currents for relief of spasm. *Arch Phys Med.* 1950;31:766-771.

19. Vodovnik L, Bowman BR, Hufford P. Effects of electrical stimulation on spinal spasticity. *Scand J Rehabil Med.* 1984;16:29.

20. Baker LL. Neuromuscular electrical stimulation in the restoration of purposeful limb movements. In Wolf SL, ed: *Clinics in Physical Therapy--Electrotherapy.* New York, NY: Churchill Livingstone; 1982:25.

21. Phillips CA. Functional electrical stimulation and lower extremity bracing for ambulation exercise of the spinal cord injured individual: A medically prescribed system. *Phys Ther.* 1989;69:842.

22. Vodovnik L, Stanic U. Functional electrical stimulation for control of locomotor systems. *Crit Rev Bioeng.* 1981;6:63-131.

23. Ralston, DJ. High voltage galvanic stimulation: can there be a "state of the art"? *Atheletic Training.* 1985;20:291.

24. Butterfield DL. The effects of high-volt pulsed current electrical stimulation on delayed-onset muscle soreness. *Journal of Athletic Training.* 1997;32:15.

25. Wolcot C. A comparison of the effects of high volt and microcurrent stimulation on delayed onset muscle soreness. *Phys Ther.* 1991;71:S117.

26. Baker LL. *Neuromuscular Electrical Stimulation: A Practical Clinical Guide.* 3rd ed. Downey, CA: Los Amigos Research and Education Institute. 1993;73-75.

27. Snyder-Mackler L, Robinson, AJ. *Clinical electrophysiology--electrotherapy and Electrophysiologic Testing.* Baltimore, Md: Williams & Wilkins; 1989:131.

28. Hunter JM, Mackin E, Callahan AD, eds. *Rehabilitation of the Hand: Surgery and Therapy.* 4th edition St. Louis, Mo: Mosby;1995.

29. Braddon RL. *Physical Medicine and Rehabilitation*. Philadelphia, PA: W.B. Saunders; 1996:23;464-486.

30. Nelson, RM, Currier DP. *Clinical Electrotherapy*. 2nd ed. Norwalk, CT: Appleton & Lange; 1991.

31. Nelson RM, Currier DP. *Clinical Electrotherapy*. 1st ed. Norwalk, CT: Appleton & Lange; 1987.

32. Scully RM, Barnes MR. *Physical Therapy*. Philadelphia, PA: Lippincott;1989;879-890.

33. Robinson, AJ, Snyder LM. *Clinical Electrophysiology*. 2nd ed. 1995;1-5:1-211.

34. Baker LL, Parker K. Neuromuscular electrical stimulation of the muscles surrounding the shoulder. *Journal of Physical Therapy*. 1986;66:12.

35. Delisa JA. *Functional Neuromuscular Stimulation, Rehabilitation Medicine: Principles and Practice*. 2nd ed. Philadelphia, PA: J.B. Lippincott; 1993.

36. Pandyan AD, Granat MH, Stott DJ. Effects of electrical stimulation on flexion contractures in the hemiplegic wrist. *Clinical Rehabilitation*. 1997;11:123-130.

37. Currier DP, et al. Effects of electrical and electromagnetic stimulation after anterior cruciate ligament reconstruction. *JOSPT*. 1993;17(4):177-184.

38. Currier DP, Mann R. Muscular strength development by electrical stimulation in healthy individuals. *Phys Ther*. 1983;63(6):915-921.

39. Doupe J, Barnes R, Kerr AS. Studies in denervation: the effect of electrical stimulation on the circulation and recovery of denervated muscle. *J Neurol Psych*. 1943;6:136.

40. Girlanda R, Dattola R, Vita G. Effect of electrotherapy on denervated muscles in rabbits: an electrophysiological and morphological study. *Exp Neurol*. 1982;77: 483.

41. Herbison GJ, Teng C-S, Gordon EE, Electrical stimulation of reinnervating rat muscle, *Arch Phys Med Rehabil*. 1973;54:156.

42. Laughmann RK, Yondas JW, Garrett TF. Strength changes in the normal quadriceps femoris muscle as a result of electrical stimulation. *Phys Ther*. 1983;63:494.

43. Schimrigk K, McLaughlin J, Gruninger W. The effect of electrical stimulation on the experimentally denervated rat muscle, *Scand J Rehabil Med*. 1977;9:55.

44. Sprilholtz N. Electrical stimulation of denervated muscle, In: Nelson RM, Currier DP. *Clinical electrotherapy*. Norwalk, CT; Appleton & Lange: 1987.

45. Sunderland S. *Nerves and Nerve Injuries*. 2nd ed. Edinburgh; Churchill Livingstone: 1978.

46. Wakim KG, Krusen FH. The influence of stimulation on the work output and endurance of denervated muscle. *Arch Phys Med Rehabil*. 1951;32:523.

47. Eriksson E, Haggmark T. Comparison of isometric muscle training and electrical stimulation supplementing isometric muscle training in the recovery after major knee ligament surgery. *Am J Sports Med*. 1979;17:169.

48. Gutmann E, Guttmann L. The effect of galvanic exercise on denervated and reinnervated muscles in the rabbit. *J Neurol Neurosurg Psychiatry*. 1944;7:7.

49. Basmajian JV, Kukulka CG, Narayan MG, Takebe K. Biofeedback treatment of foot-drop after stroke compared with standard rehabilitation technique: effects on voluntary control and strength; *Arch Phys Med Rehabil*. 1975;56:231.

50. Currier DP, Mann R. Muscular strength development by electrical stimulation in healthy individuals. *Phys Ther*. 1985;63:915.

51. Cranstam B, Larsson LE. Electrical stimulation in patients with spasticity. *Electroencephalogr Clin Neurophysiol Soc Proc*. 1975;38:214.

52. Levine MG, Knott M, Kabat H. Relaxation of spasticity by electrical stimulation of antagonist muscles. *Arch Phys Med*. 1952;33:668.

53. Alfieri V. Electrical treatment of spasticity- reflex tonic activity in hemiplegic patients and selected specific electrostimulation. *Scand J Rehab Med*. 1982;14:177.

54. Fulbright JS. Electrical stimulation to reduce chronic toe- flexor hypertonicity- A case report; *Phys Ther*. 1984;64:523.

55. Vodovnik L, Bowmann BR, Hufford P. Effects of electrical stimulation on spinal spasticity. *Scand J Rehabil Med*. 1984;16:29.

56. Cybulski GR, Penn RD, Jeager RJ. Lower extremity functional neuromuscular stimulation in cases of spinal cord injury. *Neurosurgery*. 1984;15:132.

57. LeDoux J, Quinones MA. An investigation of the use of percutaneous electrical stimulation in muscle reeducation. *Phys Ther.* 1981;61:678.

58. Cranstam B, Larsson L-E, Prevec TS. improvement of gait following functional electrical stimulation. *Scand J Rehabil Med.* 1977;9:7.

59. Merletti R, Zilaschi F, Latella D, et al. A control study of muscle force recovery in hemiparetic patients during treatment with functional electrical stimulation. *Scand J Rehabil Med.* 1978;10: 147.

60. Wienstein MV, Gordon A. The use of faradism in the rehabilitation of hemiplegics. *Phys Ther Rev.* 1974;31: 515.

61. Baker LL, Bowman Br, McNeal DR. Effects of wave form on comfort during neuromuscular electrical stimulation. *Clin Orthop.* 1988;223:75.

62. Delitto A, Rose SJ. Comparative comfort of three wave forms used in electrically eliciting quadriceps femoris muscle contractions. *Phys Ther.* 1986;66:1704.

63. Moritani T, DeVries, HA. Neural factors versus Hypertrophy in the time course of muscle strength gain. *Am J Phys Med.* 1979;58:115.

64. Fleury M Lagasse P. Influence of functional electrical stimulation training on premotor and motor reaction time. *Percept Motor Skills.* 1979;48:387.

65. Currier DP, Mann R. Muscular strength development by electrical stimulation in healthy individuals. *Phys Ther.* 1983;63:915.

66. Griffin JW. Reduction of chronic postraumatic hand edema: A comparison of high voltage pulsed current, intermittent pneumatic compression, and placebo treatments. *Phys Ther.* 1990;70:279.

67. Mohr T. The effect of high volt galvanic stimulation on quadriceps femoris muscle torque. *J Orthop Sports Phys Ther.* 1986;7:314.

68. Walker DC, Currier DP, Threlkeld AJ. Effects of high voltage pulsed electrical stimulation on blood flow. *Phys Ther.* 1988;68:481.

69. Alon, G. "Microcurrent": Subliminal electric stimulation. Does the research support its clinical use? *Sports Medicine Update.* 1993;9:8.

70. Low J, Reed A. *Electrotherapy Explained, Principles and practice.* London: Butterworth Heinemann; 1992:84-85.

71. Ferguson ACB, Granat MH. Evaluation of functional electrical stimulation for an incomplete spinal cord injured patient. *Physiotherapy.* 1992;78(4):253-256.

72. Benton, LA, et al: *Functional Electrical Stimulation—A Practical Clinical Guide.* 2nd ed. Downey, CA; Rancho Los Amigos Rehabilitation Engineering Center: 1981,1-10.

73. *Electrotherapeutic Terminology in Physical Therapy. Section on Clinical Electrophysiology.* Alexandria, VA; American Physical Therapy Association: 1990.

74. Baker LL, Parker, K, and Sanderson D. Neuromuscular electrical stimulation for the head-injured patient. *Phys Ther.* 1983;63(12).

75. Baker LL, Parker K. Neuromuscular electrical stimulation of the muscles surrounding the shoulder. *Phys Ther.* 1986;66.

76 Baker LL. Electrical stimulation of wrist and fingers for hemiplegic patients. *Phys Ther.* 1979;59:1495.

77. Alfieri V. Electrical treatment of spasticity. *Scand J Rehabil Med.* 1984;16:29.

78. Gordon T, Mao J. Muscle atrophy and procedures for training after spinal cord injury. *Phys Ther.* 1994;74:50.

Manufacturers of Electrical Stimulation Devices:

The following manufacturers have assisted in the preparation of the chapters on electrotherapy and neuromuscular electrical stimulation through their contribution of materials and information. Many of the manufacturers have information, manuals, and treatment protocols specific to their equipment which is available to the clinician. Therapists are recommended to contact the companies directly or to contact their regional sales representative.

Chatanooga Group Inc., 4717 Adams Road, PO Box 489 Hixson, TN 37343-0489

Dynatronics, 7030 Park Centre Drive, Salt Lake City, UT 84121

Electro-Med Health Industries, 11601 Biscayne Blvd. Suite 200-A, North Miami, FL 33181-3151

Empi, Inc., 1275 Grey Fox Road, St. Paul, MN 55112-6989

Mettler Electronics Corp., 1333 So. Claudina Street, Anaheim, CA 92805

Rich-Mar Corp., PO Box 879, Inola, OK 74036

Appendix

Guidelines for Electrode Placement

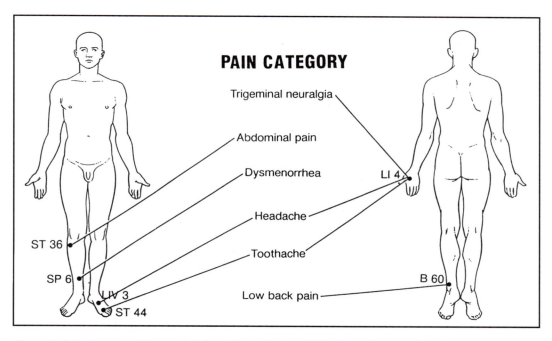

PAIN CATEGORY

Figure A-1. Basic acupuncture points for pain syndromes distant from the site of pain. Reprinted with permission from Empi, Inc., St. Paul, Minnesota.

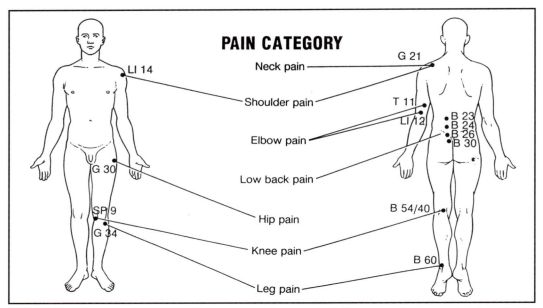

Figure A-2. Basic acupuncture points for pain syndromes which lie on or adjacent to the site of pain. Reprinted with permission from Empi, Inc., St. Paul, Mn.

Figure A-3 (A-D). Electrode placement patterns. (A) Crossed method. Reprinted with permission from Empi, Inc., St. Paul, Mn.

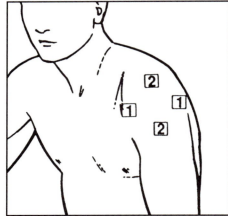

Figure A-3 (B). Bracketed method. Reprinted with permission from Empi, Inc., St. Paul, Mn.

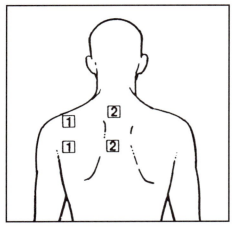

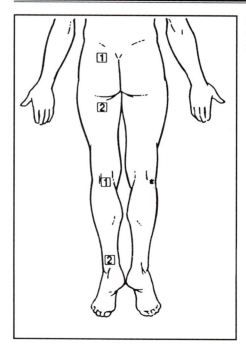

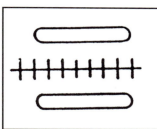

Figure A-3 (C). Unilateral, linear and overlapping with distal point. Reprinted with permission from Empi, Inc., St. Paul, Mn.

Figure A-3 (D). Parallel; on either side of a scar or incision. Reprinted with permission from Empi, Inc., St. Paul, Mn.

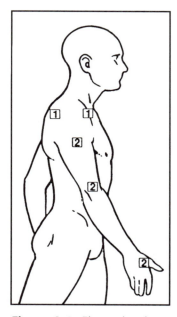

Figure A-4. Electrode placement suggestions for shoulder pain. Reprinted with permission from Empi, Inc., St. Paul, Mn.

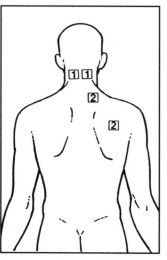

Figure A-5. Electrode placement for scapular pain with headache symptoms. Reprinted with permission from Empi, Inc., St. Paul., Mn.

Figure A-6. Electrode placement for combination shoulder and scapular pain.Reprinted with permission from Empi, Inc., St. Paul, Mn.

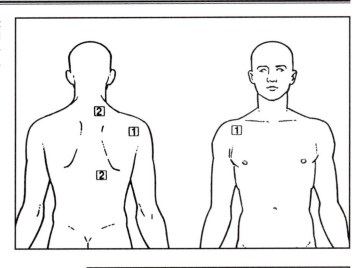

Figure A-7. Electrode placement suggestion for shoulder pain. Place one electrode directly above posterior axillary fold below spine of scapula and the other at upper trapezius (directly above superior angle of scapula); place one electrode at anterior/inferior aspect of AC joint and the other at the lateral aspect of elbow crease in depression when elbow is flexed. Reprinted with permission from Empi, Inc., St. Paul, Mn.

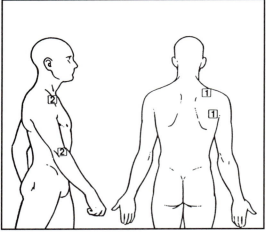

Index